A PRIMER ON AMNIOTIC MEMBRANE REGENERATIVE HEALING

Thomas J. Koob, PhD
Chief Scientific Officer

Conan S. Young, PhD
Director of Research

Jeremy J. Lim, PhD
Senior Biomedical Engineer

Kathryn Chinn
Biomedical Engineer

Michelle Massee
Manager of Biomedical Research

Marissa Carter, PhD
Consulting Statistician

Randall Spencer
Vice President of Clinical Innovation

David Mason, MD
Vice President of Medical Affairs for Clinical Practice

Donald Fetterolf, MD, MBA, FACP
Chief Medical Officer

Reviewers:
William W. Li, MD
President and Medical Director, The Angiogenesis Foundation

Mary Pat Moyer, PhD
*Chief Executive Officer and Chief Science Officer,
INCELL Corporation, LLC*

MiMedx Group, Inc.
1775 West Oak Commons Court NE
Marietta, GA 30062
(770) 651-9100

MiMedx/Color House Graphics
3505 Eastern Ave SE
Grand Rapids, MI 49508
www.colorhousegraphics.com/

A Primer on Amniotic Membrane Regenerative Healing /
Thomas J. Koob, PhD, et al. — 3rd ed.
ISBN 978-0-692-51694-2

TABLE OF CONTENTS

PREFACE

Since MiMedx introduced amniotic membrane tissue allografts in 2006, there has been a steady increase in the utilization of this tissue. The use of these allografts in advanced wound care has escalated very rapidly since 2012, and its utilization in certain surgical procedures has steadily increased since 2013. When any new technology with significant promise escalates this rapidly, there are numerous issues that develop particularly when the technology is complex both scientifically and clinically. The chance for misinformation and pseudoscience is heightened, and this is a disservice to the clinicians and scientists who are attempting to substantiate the attributes of the new technology.

In 1968, I was fortunate enough to be involved in a rapidly emerging new technology which was given the name of Advanced Composite Materials. These materials were being examined for use on aircraft structures, and their promise drew focus from numerous corporate entities and the Air Force Materials Laboratory. Because the composite technology was quite complex and very difficult for structural engineers to analyze, I coauthored a Primer with two other industry participants on the science and engineering analytics of those complex materials. The Primer was well received because it provided this emerging industry adequate reference material that was easily understood by most participants, including engineers, scientists, and management.

Because of this previous experience, I felt strongly that the same type of Primer was necessary due to the rapid growth of amniotic membrane allografts. Therefore, I gave the assignment to the MiMedx scientists and clinicians to develop this Primer. In addition, we asked certain consultants to participate. We thank both the MiMedx staff and these consultants for this exceptional manuscript.

As a member of the American Academy of Engineering, I understand the necessity and requirements for scientific rigor. Since this amnion processing technology has developed quite rapidly, I have been quite concerned about the misinformation and pseudoscience that has developed as some organizations rushed to place their version of amniotic allografts in the market place. I hope this Primer will help bring some discipline to the process, and therefore, assist clinicians in making their assessments as to the attributes of these allografts that make them more effective than conventional therapies.

We believe the information contained in this Primer will be very beneficial to clinicians, scientists, as well as other individuals who are attempting to understand the potential benefits and uses of amniotic membrane allografts. Truly, amniotic membrane does offer some unique qualities and possibilities to enhance healing, reduce scar tissue formation, and modulate inflammation. However, there must be a discipline associated with bringing these new products and technology into commercialization.

We are offering this Primer to healthcare professionals to help educate and bring order and discipline to the development and use of this promising tissue and technology. This Primer should clarify numerous issues in terms of the healing process, the modes of action of these allografts, and the basis for demonstrating clinical safety and efficacy for amniotic membrane allografts. I hope you will appreciate our motives for developing this book, and we will certainly welcome constructive criticism.

Parker H. "Pete" Petit
Chairman and CEO
MiMedx Group, Inc.
August 18, 2015

TABLE OF ABBREVIATIONS

ABBREVIATION	DEFINITION
AAALAC	Association for Assessment and Accreditation of Laboratory Animal Care
ADM	acellular dermal matrix
ADSC	adipose-derived stem cell
AE	adverse event
Ang	angiogenin
Ang-1/2	angiopoietin-1/2
BDNF	brain-derived neurotrophic factor
bFGF	basic fibroblast growth factor
BLA	Biologics License Application
BLC	B lymphocyte chemoattractant
BMP	bone morphogenetic protein
CBER	FDA Center for Biologics Evaluation and Research
CCL	C-C motif chemokine ligand
CD	cluster of differentiation
CDER	FDA Center for Drug Evaluation and Research
cDNA	complementary deoxyribonucleic acid
CDRH	FDA Center for Devices and Radiological Health
CFR	Code of Federal Regulations
cGMP	current Good Manufacturing Practices
cGTP	current Good Tissue Practices
CMS	Centers for Medicare & Medicaid Services
CMV	cytomegalovirus
CONSORT	Consolidated Standards of Reporting Trials
CRF	Case Report Form
CTA	Clinical Trial Agreement
CTGF	connective tissue growth factor
CXCL	C-X-C motif chemokine ligand
DFU	diabetic foot ulcer
dHACM	dehydrated human amnion/chorion membrane
DMSO	dimethylsulfoxide
DNA	deoxyribonucleic acid
ECM	extracellular matrix
EGF	epidermal growth factor

ABBREVIATION	DEFINITION
EG-VEGF	endocrine gland-derived vascular endothelial growth factor
ELISA	enzyme-linked immunosorbent assay
EMR	electronic medical record
FACIT	fibril associate collagen with interrupted triple helices
FDA	Food and Drug Administration
FDR	false discovery rate
FGF	fibroblast growth factor
FWA	Federal Wide Assurance
FWER	familywise error rate
GAG	glycosaminoglycan
GCP	Good Clinical Practices
GCSF	granulocyte colony-stimulating factor
GDF	growth differentiation factor
GFP	green fluorescent protein
GH	growth hormone
GM-CSF	granulocyte macrophage colony-stimulating factor
GMP	Good Manufacturing Practices
GTP	Good Tissue Practices
H&E	hematoxylin and eosin
HB-EGF	heparin binding epidermal growth factor-like growth factor
HCF	human cardiac fibroblast
HCT/P	Human Cell, Tissue, and Cellular and Tissue-Based Product
HDF	human dermal fibroblast
HGF	hepatocyte growth factor
HHS	Department of Health and Human Services
HIV	human immunodeficiency virus
HLA	human leukocyte antigen
HPC	hematopoietic progenitor cell
HSC	hematopoietic stem cell
HTLV	human T-lymphotropic virus
I-309	C-C motif chemokine ligand 1 (CCL1)
IACUC	Institutional Animal Care and Use Committee
ICF	Informed Consent Form
ICH	International Conference on Harmonization
IDE	Investigational Device Exemption

ABBREVIATION	DEFINITION
IEC	Independent/Institutional Ethics Committee
IFN	interferon
Ig	immunoglobulin
IGF	insulin-like growth factor
IGFBP	insulin-like growth factor binding protein
ICH	International Conference on Harmonization
IL	interleukin
IL-Ra	interleukin receptor antagonist
IND	Investigational New Drug
iNOS	inducible nitric oxide synthase
IP	interferon gamma-induced protein
IRB	Institutional Review Board
ITT	intention to treat
JAPMA	Journal of the American Podiatric Medical Association
KGF	keratinocyte growth factor
LAR	legally authorized representative
LPS	lipopolysaccharide
MCP	monocyte chemotactic protein
MCSF	macrophage colony-stimulating factor
MDC	macrophage-derived chemokine
MHC	major histocompatibility complex
MIG	monokine induced by gamma interferon
MIP	macrophage inflammatory protein
MLCT	multi-layer compression therapy
MMC	Mitomycin C
MMP	matrix metalloproteinases
mRNA	messenger ribonucleic acid
MSC	mesenchymal stromal/stem cell
MT-MMP	membrane type matrix metalloproteinases
NDA	New Drug Application
NDA	nondisclosure agreement
NIH	National Institutes of Health
NGF	nerve growth factor
NK	natural killer

ABBREVIATION	DEFINITION
OCT	optimal cutting temperature
OHRP	Office for Human Research Protections
OIG	Office of the Inspector General
OPG	osteoprotegerin
PARC	pulmonary and activation-regulated chemokine
PCR	polymerase chain reaction
pDC	plasmacytoid dendritic cell
PDGF	platelet-derived growth factor
pen/strep	penicillin/streptomycin
PlGF	placental growth factor
PMA	Premarket Approval
RANTES	regulated on activation, normal T cell expressed and secreted
RCT	randomized controlled trial
RNA	ribonucleic acid
ROC	receiver operating characteristic
ROS	reactive oxygen species
RT	reverse transcription
SAE	serious adverse event
Sca	stem cell antigen
SCF	stem cell factor
SDF	stromal cell derived factor
SIS	small intestinal submucosa
SLRP	small leucine-rich proteoglycan
SMC	smooth muscle cell
SOC	Standard of Care
SVF	stromal vascular fraction
TARC	thymus and activation-regulated chemokine
TGF	transforming growth factor
TIMP	tissue inhibitor of metalloproteinases
TLR	toll-like receptor
TNF	tumor necrosis factor
VEGF	vascular endothelial growth factor
VLU	venous leg ulcer

DEFINITIONS OF FREQUENTLY USED TERMS

TERM	DEFINITION
Absorbance	Amount of light that is taken up by a sample, and not transmitted through the sample
Adaptive immunity	Immune response formed from immunological memory after an initial response
Adipocyte	Fat cell
Adipose derived stem cell (ADSC)	Type of mesenchymal stem cells found in fat tissue
Allogeneic	From a different individual of the same species
Allograft	Tissue graft from a different individual of the same species
Amnion	Innermost layer of the amniotic membrane
Amniotic membrane	Placental membrane, comprised of the amnion and chorion layers, which makes up the amniotic sac
Amniotic sac	Sac which holds the developing fetus and amniotic fluid and is comprised of the amniotic membrane
Amniotic tissue	Placental tissue that composes the amniotic membrane, including amnion and chorion
Angiogenesis	Formation of new blood vessels from pre-existing vessels
Antibody	Protein produced by plasma cells during the adaptive immune response to bind and identify specific foreign molecules
Apoptosis	Process of programmed cell death
Assay	Analytical procedure to measure the presence, quantity, or activity of a target component or function
Autocrine	Refers to signals that are released from and bind to receptors on the same cell
Autograft	Tissue graft from the same patient
Autologous	From the same individual
B cell	Lymphocyte white blood cell of the adaptive immune response
Basal medium	Culture medium without growth supplements
Basophil	Granulocyte white blood cell
Blinded	In clinical trials, prevention of a tested individual from knowing what treatment is given or the treating clinician from knowing what treatment was applied
Blood vessel	Tubular structure that carries blood throughout the body
Cardiomyocyte	Muscle cell of the heart
Cell	Smallest structural and functional unit of an organism
Chemoattractant	Chemical that induces a cell to migrate toward it
Chemokine	Cytokines that recruit cell migration through directed chemotaxis
Chemotaxis	Migration of cells in response to a chemical stimulus

TERM	DEFINITION
Chondrocyte	Cartilage cell
Chorion	Outermost layer of the amniotic membrane
Chronic wound	Wound that fails to heal in an orderly and timely manner, often greater than 3 months
Clinical trial	Research studies to test how well new medical approaches work in people, such as better ways to prevent, screen for, diagnose, or treat a disease
Collagen	Main structural protein in connective tissues
Complete medium	Culture medium containing growth supplements
Confluence	Proportion of surface area covered by adherent cells
Control	Known sample that is evaluated to determine the accuracy of analytical results
Controlled	In clinical trials, when assignment of subjects is controlled by a process that fairly assigns potential candidates and prevents self-selection or similar biases from affecting the randomization process
Cryopreservation	Storage by freezing
Culture medium	Liquid designed to support growth of cells
Cytokine	Signaling protein that is secreted by cells and affects the behavior of other cells
Decellularization	Tissue processing method that removes cellular material
Degranulation	Cellular process that releases signaling molecules from secretory vesicles
Dehydration	Removal of water/moisture
Dendritic cell	Antigen-presenting white blood cell of the adaptive immune responses
Deoxyribonucleic acid (DNA)	Genetic material in organisms
Dermis	Inner base layer of the skin
Dynamic reciprocity	Bidirectional interaction between cells and their surrounding microenvironments
Efficacy	Capacity to produce a beneficial or therapeutic effect
Elastin	Fibrous protein with elastic, spring-like properties
Enzyme-linked immunosorbent assay (ELISA)	Analytical assay that uses antibodies and a reporter molecule or enzyme to quantify a molecular concentration
Endocrine	Refers to signals that are released into the bloodstream and bind receptors on cells that are distant in the body
Endogenous	From the same organism, tissue, or cell
Endothelial cell	Cell that forms the inner layer of blood vessels
Enzyme	Substance that acts as a catalyst to accelerate a chemical reaction
Eosinophil	Granulocyte white blood cell

TERM	DEFINITION
Epidermis	Outer layer of the skin
Epithelial cell	Cell that lines the major cavities of the body and makes up the outer surface of the body
Extracellular matrix (ECM)	Proteins and polysaccharides secreted by cells that provide structural and biochemical support
Extravasation	Process by which leukocytes migrate across blood vessel walls into tissues
FDA Form 1571	Investigational New Drug (IND) application form
FDA Form 1572	Statement of Investigators for Investigational New Drug (IND) application
Fibril	Fine fiber
Fibrin	Fibrous protein involved in clotting of blood
Fibroblast	Connective tissue cell that synthesizes extracellular matrix
Fibrocyte	Inactive form of a fibroblast
Fibronectin	Glycoprotein involved in cell adhesion
Flow cytometry	Microfluidic analytical technique to count cells and detect cellular biomarkers
Fluorescence	Light emitted from a sample following excitation
Free radicals	Reactive molecule that has an unpaired valence electron
Gene expression	Process by which genetic information is translated from DNA to mRNA to protein
Glycoprotein	Proteins that contain covalently bound oligosaccharide chains
Granulation	Formation of disorganized connective tissue to fill a healing wound
Granulocyte	Category of white blood cells including neutrophils, eosinophils, basophils, and mast cells
Green fluorescent protein (GFP)	Protein derived from jellyfish that exhibits green fluorescence
Growth factor (GF)	Signaling protein that is secreted by cells and capable of stimulating cellular growth
Growth medium	Culture medium containing growth supplements
Hematopoietic stem cell	Multipotent cell that can differentiate into all other blood cells
Hemostasis	Process which causes blood to clot
Heparin	Compound that inhibits blood coagulation
Histamine	Compound released by cells in response to injury or allergic reaction
Histology	Study of microscopy anatomy of cells and tissues through section and staining
Hormone	Substance produced by glands and transported by the circulatory system
Human leukocyte antigen (HLA)	Set of cell surface molecules that regulate the immune system in humans; comprised of 3 classes of molecules: Class I, Class II, Class III

TERM	DEFINITION
Hyaluronan	Polysaccharide chain widely distributed throughout connective, epithelial, and neural tissues
Hypoxia	Deficiency of oxygen
Immunomodulation	Modification of the immune response
Immunologically privileged	Ability to not elicit an inflammatory immune response
In vitro	Latin for "in glass"; refers to in the laboratory
In vivo	Latin for "within the living"; refers to within living organisms
Inflammation	Biological response of the immune system to harmful stimuli, such as damage or infection
Innate immunity	Immune response that nonspecifically responds to foreign pathogens
Interleukin (IL)	Cytokine involved in cell signaling of the immune system, inflammation, and tissue repair
Keratinocyte	Cell of the epidermis
Laminin	Structural protein found in basal lamina of basement membranes
Leukocyte	White blood cell
Level of evidence	Ranking of clinical trials based on strength and reliability
Ligand	Molecule that binds and forms a complex with a receptor, triggering a signal
Lipopolysaccharide (LPS)	Molecular component of bacterial cell wall
Luminescence	Light emitted from a sample without requiring excitation
Lymphocytes	Category of white blood cells including T cells and B cells of the adaptive immune response and natural killer cells of the innate immune response
Macrophage	White blood cell that differentiates from monocytes and is part of both the innate and adaptive immune responses
Major histocompatibility complex (MHC)	Set of cell surface molecules involved in regulating the immune system and recognizing foreign substances; in humans, the complex is also called human leukocyte antigen (HLA)
Mast cell	Granulocyte white blood cell
Matrix metalloproteinases (MMPs)	Enzymes that degrade extracellular matrix
Mesenchymal stromal/stem cell (MSC)	Multipotent cell that can assist tissue repair, modulate the immune response, and differentiate into various types of mesenchymal tissue lineages (e.g., bone, cartilage, fat) and other cell types under appropriate conditions
Migration	Movement from one location to another
Mitomycin C (MMC)	Chemical that cross links DNA; used to inhibit cell division and proliferation
Mitosis	Process of cellular division and replication
Monocyte	White blood cell that differentiates into macrophages

TERM	DEFINITION
Myoblast	Progenitor cell that becomes a muscle cell
Myocyte	Muscle cell
Natural killer (NK) cell	Cytotoxic white blood cell of the innate immune system
Necrosis	Cellular injury that results in cell death
Negative control	Sample group in which no response or only a baseline response is expected
Neutrophil	Granulocyte white blood cell
Nucleus	Organelle containing genetic material of cells
Organ	Collection of tissues joined in a structural unit to perform a common function
Osteoblast	Cell that synthesizes bone
Osteoclast	Cell that degrades bone
Osteocyte	Bone cell that is embedded in mineralized matrix
Parabiosis	Anatomical joining of two individuals
Paracrine	Refers to signals that are released and binds receptors on a different cell
Pericyte	Cells that wrap around and stabilize vascular tubes
Phagocytosis	Cell eating; process by which a cell engulfs and digests pathogens and tissue debris
Placenta	Organ that supports and connects a developing fetus to the maternal uterine wall
Plasmacytoid dendritic cell (pDC)	Specialized white blood cell of the innate immune system
Plate reader	Instrument used to quantify absorbance, fluorescence, or luminescence of light from a microplate
Platelet	Component of blood whose function is to stop bleeding
Polymerase chain reaction (PCR)	Molecular biology technique that rapidly amplifies DNA across several orders of magnitude using enzymes, gene specific primers, and thermocycles
Positive control	Sample group in which a known response is expected
Proliferation	Increase in cell number through cell division
Proteins	Molecules composed of chains of amino acids; may be complexed with sugars (glycoproteins) or lipids (lipoproteins)
Proteoglycan	Protein with covalently bound polysaccharide chains called glycosaminoglycans
Randomized	In clinical trials, when patients are placed into treatment or control groups by random assignment
Reactive oxygen species (ROS)	Chemically reactive molecules containing oxygen

TERM	DEFINITION
Receptor	Protein on or in a cell that binds chemical signals in the form of ligands
Recruitment	Chemotactic migration of cells, often from the bloodstream or surrounding tissue, toward a chemoattractant
Remodeling	Reorganization of tissue
Replicates	Repetition of an experimental condition to estimate the variability within a sample group or experimental response
Reverse transcription (RT)	Generation of complementary DNA from a messenger RNA template
Ribonucleic acid (RNA)	Molecule involved in coding, decoding, regulation, and expression of genes
Serum	Cell culture growth supplement derived as a liquid from coagulated blood
Sham	Surgical control in which a similar treatment of procedure is performed while omitting a key therapeutic element of the treatment under investigation
Smooth muscle cell (SMC)	Cell of involuntary non-striated muscle
Standard curve	Graph that shows a relationship between two known quantities; used to determine the value of an unknown quantity
Standard of Care (SOC)	Generally accepted form of treatment for a certain medical condition
Stem cell	Cell that is capable of self-renewal and can form other specialized cell types through differentiation
Steroid	Substance composed of a specific carbon ring structure that can signal to cells
Subcutaneous	Under the skin
System	Group of organs that work together to perform a common set of functions
T cell	Lymphocyte white blood cell of the adaptive immune response
Tissue	Collection of similar cells from the same origin that perform a specific function
Tissue extract	Solution which contains soluble factors that are released from a tissue into the surrounding liquid
Tissue inhibitor of matrix metallopro-teinases (TIMP)	Molecules that inhibit activity of matrix metalloproteinases
Toll-like receptor (TLR)	Important cell surface marker of innate cell responses
Trypsin	Digestive enzyme that degrades proteins, often used to detach cells
Ulcer	Sore that developed on a bodily membrane, such as the skin
Vascularization	Formation of blood vessels
Vasoconstriction	Narrowing of blood vessels
Vasodilation	Widening of blood vessels
Xenograft	Tissue graft from an animal of a different species

CHAPTER 1

TISSUE REGENERATION AND HEALING

Tissue regeneration has become the new standard for healing and repair. The goal of tissue regeneration is to repair and replace damaged or diseased tissue with healthy tissue that is fully functional, free of scar tissue, and completely replicates the healthy, pre-injury tissue. In contrast, the current state of tissue healing or repair often results in tissue that may look, feel, or function differently from healthy tissue. While healing and repair are often sufficient to remedy the root symptoms of injury, full tissue regeneration remains to be the goal when treating damaged tissues.

Tissues are primarily composed of cells and extracellular matrix. Cells are the biological building blocks of tissue. They maintain the function of the tissue by synthesizing proteins or metabolizing waste. Single cells communicate with one another and respond to stimuli in their surrounding environments. Cells secrete and maintain extracellular matrix (ECM) which is the structural component of tissues. Cells interact with each other and the ECM through direct contact as well as soluble signaling molecules, including cytokines, growth factors, hormones, steroids, enzymes, and other chemicals. These signals stimulate a chain reaction or cascade which alters cell behavior, both in the releasing cell itself, as well as other neighboring cells of a tissue. Cells (for example, cardiomyocytes) are organized to function together with their structural matrix as a tissue (e.g., cardiac muscle); tissues compose organs (e.g., heart) which interact together as an organ system (e.g., circulatory system) to control bodily function, as shown in Figure 1. These hierarchical components and systems require remarkable coordination of signals and responses to sustain life, respond to injury, and stimulate a healing response. Healing involves coordinated responses by numerous cell types from throughout the body to regenerate injured tissues. Further discussion of the cell types, extracellular matrix components, and molecular signals that play roles in healing are discussed in detail in Chapters 3, 4, and 5 of this Primer.

Cell	Tissue	Organ	System

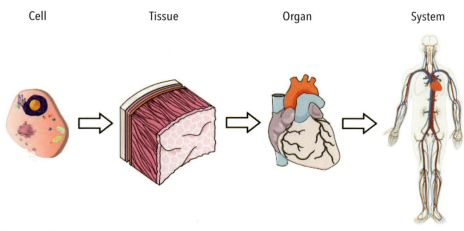

Figure 1. Cells compose tissues, tissues compose organs, organs compose systems, and systems control and maintain the body and support growth and healing.[a]

1.1 HEALING

The human body possesses a remarkable capacity to heal. Following tissue damage or disease, the body's immune response coordinates a sequence of events to fight off harmful diseases or infections and repair the damaged tissue. The body's most immediate concern in response to injury is to close the wound to stop bleeding and prevent infection. While scar tissue may form as a byproduct of rapid healing, scar tissue may be remodeled over time under the proper conditions.

1.1.1 HEMOSTASIS

Following injury, a wound immediately enters the process of *hemostasis*, where the blood vessels clot in order to stop bleeding. During hemostasis, blood vessels constrict to slow blood flow and reduce blood loss. Platelets then aggregate to form a plug to stop bleeding, and blood coagulates to form a fibrin clot which reinforces the platelet plug. This process is controlled through complex molecular signals from the rupture of surrounding blood vessels. During this process, platelets also undergo *degranulation*, where platelets release their contents into the blood stream and surrounding tissue matrix, releasing a wide array of growth factors, chemokines, as well as vasodilators. Growth factors and cytokines released during platelet degranulation include platelet-derived growth factor (PDGF), transforming growth factor β (TGF-β), fibroblast

[a] Figure adapted from https://openclipart.org/detail/157339/celula-eucariotica (Public domain), http://www.servier.com/Powerpoint-image-bank (Servier Medical Art By Servier, Heart_physiology, Creative Commons Attribution 3.0 Unported), and http://commons.wikimedia.org/wiki/File:Circulatory_System_no_tags.svg (Public domain).

growth factor (FGF), insulin-like growth factor (IGF), vascular endothelial growth factor (VEGF), epidermal growth factor (EGF), keratinocyte growth factor (KGF), connective tissue growth factor (CTGF), tumor necrosis factor (TNF), and interleukin (IL) molecules such as IL-1 and IL-8.[1] These regulatory molecules activate fibroblasts and stimulate the local healing response.

Following hemostasis which typically last several minutes, the physiological healing response is traditionally considered to progress through 3 stages of healing in response to injury: 1) inflammation, 2) proliferation, and 3) remodeling, as shown in Figure 2.

Normal Wound Healing

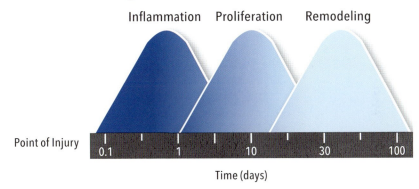

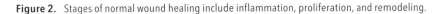

Figure 2. Stages of normal wound healing include inflammation, proliferation, and remodeling.

1.1.2 INFLAMMATION

The first stage of inflammation begins immediately following injury and may last over the course of hours to days. Following injury, damaged cells and degranulating platelets immediately release cytokines, chemokines, and regulatory molecules that stimulate inflammation and the healing response. Inflammation typically involves swelling, where fluid accumulates in the injured and surrounding tissue, causing the injured area to become red and sensitive. This inflammation occurs as white blood cells, also called leukocytes, infiltrate the injured tissue. White blood cells are present in the blood, where they circulate throughout the body via blood vessels. Following injury, cells and platelets release chemoattractants, which are chemicals that attract leukocyte migration, into the wound. These chemoattractants including chemokines recruit leukocytes to migrate across the blood vessel wall into the wound, through a process called leukocyte extravasation. Since blood vessel walls are composed of endothelial cells, leukocyte extravasation is regulated by the expression of adhesion molecules on the endothelial cells. In the wound, the migrating and local inflammatory cells are responsible for removing necrotic tissue and debris, fighting infection, breaking down the clot, recruiting new fibroblasts to migrate into the wound and aid repair, and promoting angiogenesis. They also release additional immunomodulatory chemicals to control the inflammatory process.

The first immune cells to respond to injury are neutrophils, mast cells, specialized dendritic cells, and monocytes. *Neutrophils* invade the wounded tissue within hours and are primarily involved in *phagocytosis*, where a cell engulfs and digests pathogens and tissue debris, and cleans the wound in response to bacterial infection and necrotic tissue.[2] This first step can be compared to surgical debridement, where inflammatory cells rather than the physician remove bacteria and necrotic tissue from the wound. Neutrophils engulf and eat bacteria and release highly reactive *free radicals* (otherwise known as reactive oxygen species or "ROS") to kill infectious agents and suppress infection.[1] ROS react by oxidizing complex biological molecules, such as proteins and DNA, rendering them non-functional in a cell and potentially leading to death of the cell. Neutrophils also release pro- and anti-inflammatory immunomodulatory *cytokines*, including TNF-α, IL-1α, IL-1β, IL-1Ra, IL-3, IL-12, interferon gamma (IFN-γ), TGF-β, granulocyte colony-stimulating factor (GCSF), macrophage colony-stimulating factor (MCSF), and granulocyte macrophage colony-stimulating factor (GM-CSF). In addition, neutrophils act to recruit more cells by secreting *chemokines* like IL-8, macrophage inflammatory protein 1α (MIP-1α), MIP-1β, and monocyte chemotactic protein 1 (MCP-1), which attract monocytes/macrophages into the wound, and *angiogenic growth factors* like vascular endothelial growth factor (VEGF) and hepatocyte growth factor (HGF), which are important for promoting the formation of new blood vessels.[3] Collectively these molecules play important roles in the healing process, where they stimulate tissue regeneration by host cells, as well as downstream effects on inflammatory cells including monocytes, granulocytes, and lymphocytes. The presence of neutrophils in the wound typically diminishes after approximately 3 days; however, neutrophils have been shown to persist in chronic wounds, suggesting that their prolonged presence may inhibit healing.

Mast cells are tissue resident granulocytes that contain granules rich in histamine and heparin. Although usually associated with an allergic response, mast cells play an important role in the initial wound and early healing responses within the first 24 hours, including inflammation and angiogenesis.[4] In the initial stages of healing, mast cells release histamine and heparin, altering blood coagulation and causing vessel leakage and fluid accumulation, which lead to the characteristic signs of acute inflammation: rubor (redness), calor (heat), tumor (swelling), and dolor (pain). Additional chemotactic mediators including IL-8, I-309, MCP-1, MIP-1α, -1β contribute to these processes, while proinflammatory cytokines including IL-1β, IL-3, IL-4, IL-6, IL-10, IL-12, IL-13, IL-16, TNF-a and growth promoting factors TGF-β, stem cell factor (SCF), nerve growth

4

factor (NGF), GM-CSF, M-CSF, PDGF, bFGF, VEGF contribute to neoangiogenesis, fibrogenesis, and re-epithelialization.[4] They may continue to be exposed to and secrete molecular mediators and proteases during remodeling and contribute to the overall healing process.[5]

Specialized plasmacytoid dendritic cells (pDCs) also respond innately through toll-like receptors (TLR) 7 and 9 to injury with a rapid and robust infiltration of pDCs that parallels the early wound infiltration by neutrophils within the first 24 hours. After responding to release of host nucleic acids from damaged tissue, they contribute to wound healing and antimicrobial action through induction of type I interferons α and β.[6]

Within the first 2 to 3 days, *monocytes* and *dendritic cells* also invade the damaged tissue, in response to chemokines including RANTES (regulated on activation, normal T cell expressed and secreted; CCL5), MIP-1α/β, I-309 (CCL1), and MCP-1, which are released by platelets and neutrophils.[7] After leaving the bloodstream and entering the damaged tissue, monocytes differentiate into *macrophages*. These macrophages are primarily responsible for engulfing foreign bodies (including infectious microbes) and damaged tissue, similar to neutrophils. However, macrophages and dendritic cells have the important function of antigen processing and presentation as part of the acquired immune response, in conjunction with T and B lymphocytes. Macrophages also play an important role in releasing chemical signals which stimulate blood vessel formation and tissue formation. Macrophages are known to secrete TGF-α, TGF-β, PDGF, IGF-I, TNF-α, IL-1, and IL-6.[2] These signals recruit mesenchymal stromal or stem cells (MSCs), fibroblasts, and lymphocytes to migrate into the wound and promote granulation and angiogenesis in the proliferation stage of healing. Macrophages also produce *reactive oxygen species* (ROS) which combat infection, and are involved in tissue remodeling through expression of matrix metalloproteinases (MMPs) and tissue inhibitors of matrix metalloproteinases (TIMPs).[2]

Activated macrophages have been shown to differentiate into two distinct phenotypes, which are referred to as the "classically activated" M1 and "alternatively activated" M2 macrophages.[8-10] These phenotypes work in concert to balance inflammation within the wounds. "Classically activated" M1 macrophages are primed by IFN-γ and activated by stimulating signals such as bacterial lipopolysaccharide (LPS).[11, 12] M1 macrophages engulf foreign pathogens, and generally promote an increase in inflammation including release of IL-1β, IL-6, IL-12, and TNF-α, as well as secretion of chemokines like IL-8, interferon gamma-induced protein 10 (IP-10)/C-X-C motif chemokine ligand 10 (CXCL10), MIP-1α, MIP-1β, and RANTES which recruit neutrophils, immature dendritic cells, natural killer cells, and activated T cells to the wound.[8-10, 13] M1 macrophages also produce MMPs-1, -2, -7, -9, -12 which enzymatically degrade ECM, including collagen, elastin, and fibronectin.[14, 15]

While M1 macrophages are generally associated with inflammation and pathogen removal, the "alternatively activated" M2 macrophages, on the other hand, are typically associated with reduction of inflammation and promotion of tissue repair.[8-10] M2 macrophages are activated in response to IL-4 or IL-13.[16, 17] M2 macrophages decrease overall inflammation and encourage tissue repair through release of anti-inflammatory factors such as IL-1Ra, IL-10, and TGF-β and chemokines such as macrophage-derived chemokine (MDC)/C-C motif chemokine 22 (CCL22), pulmonary and activation-regulated chemokine (PARC)/CCL18, and thymus and activation-regulated chemokine (TARC)/CCL17.[18-23] M2 macrophages also assist the repair process by secreting fibrogenic and angiogenic growth factors, such as PDGF, IGF, TGF-β, basic fibroblast growth factor (bFGF), TGF-α, and VEGF.[24, 25] These molecules secreted by M2 macrophages contribute toward the resolution of inflammation and promotion of wound repair.

M1 macrophage phenotype can be measured through inducible nitric oxide synthase (iNOS) activity, and M2 phenotype can be measured using arginase activity.[26-28] Both of these macrophage phenotypes work together to regulate a reparative immune response, not alone or in isolation; therefore, the balance of M1 and M2 activity (or iNOS:arginase activity) is an important marker of the healing response and the relative contributions of the two macrophage phenotypes. A predominance of M2 over M1 macrophages may suggest the wound is proceeding normally along an acute healing trajectory, while a predominance of the M1 phenotype for a prolonged period of time may suggest ongoing, chronic inflammation at the wound site.[29]

Lymphocytes are a class of white blood cells that include T cells, B cells, and natural killer (NK) cells. Of these, *NK cells* are correlated with an early presence during inflammation and response modulation, whereas *T cells* play the largest role in the healing process. T cells peak in the wound after 7 days.[2] These T lymphocytes recognize "non-self" antigens, work in concert with antigen presenting cells, and mount a response to eliminate foreign pathogens or rogue cells. T cells can be classified as cytotoxic, helper, and suppressor T cells. Cytotoxic T cells, which carry the surface marker cluster of differentiation 8 (CD8), bind major histocompatibility complex I (MHC I) expressed on the surface of virus-infected cells and kill them. Cytotoxic T cells are generally believed to downregulate repair processes.[30] Helper T-cells, which are positive for CD4, are activated by binding MHC II on antigen presenting cells, where they activate and regulate T and B cells.[2] Helper T cells are considered to promote tissue regeneration. This balance of helper and cytotoxic T cells is required to regulate fibrous tissue growth and to promote tissue repair and remodeling through angiogenic and fibrogenic factors.

The relative presence of cells involved in inflammation, healing, and repair is depicted in Figure 3.

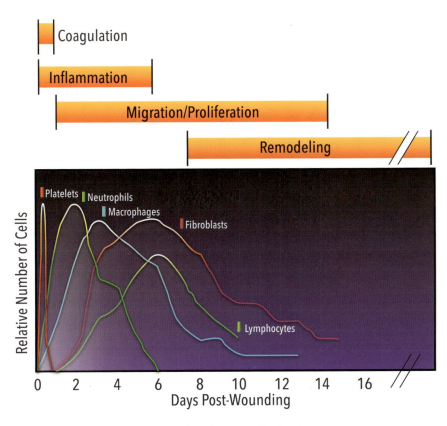

Figure 3. Cell populations in a wound throughout the stages of healing.[2]

1.1.3 IMPORTANCE OF INFLAMMATION IN HEALING

While inflammation is often viewed in a negative connotation, inflammation is actually an essential component of the healing process. Inflammation is commonly associated with pain, swelling, heat, and redness; however, these effects are the body's natural response to injury and extravasation, as blood and white blood cells move out of the vessels into the tissue and stimulate the repair process.[2, 31] Therefore it is important to understand that even though certain molecular signals are traditionally identified as *pro-inflammatory* molecules, they are also critical molecules to support *tissue regeneration* through stimulation of reparative cells. In contrast, only persistent inflammation, as seen in chronic wounds, can lead to tissue damage and prevent progression through the healing process. Molecular mediators, extracellular matrix, nutritional environment, pH, and other factors all play roles in chronic inflammation. Therefore, the key to promoting tissue regeneration within these chronically inflamed wounds is to restore homeostasis by altering the balance of immunomodulatory cytokines and other elements of the microenvironment in order to reset the healing trajectory from one of chronic inflammation to one of acute healing to allow the wound to progress through the natural healing process.

Modulation of inflammation, rather than simply reduction of inflammation, is an important concept in facilitating the body's natural ability to heal and repair from injury. Broad scale suppression of inflammation systemically or locally may inhibit the body's physiological healing response by reducing the presence and activity of reparative cells in the wounds. Modulation of inflammation through a proper balance of pro- and anti-inflammatory signals, however, is critical to facilitate the natural inflammation stage of wound healing, while subsequently propelling the healing trajectory out of a chronically inflamed state into an acute healing response.

1.1.4 CELL PROLIFERATION

The proliferation stage of healing may occur over the course of days to weeks. During this phase, inflammation begins to subside as neutrophils and macrophages decrease in number within the wound after having cleared the wound bed of foreign bodies and necrotic tissue, and then *resident cells* in the tissue, such as fibroblasts in dermal tissue and stem cells, *migrate* and *proliferate* to replace the damaged tissue. These cells deposit *extracellular matrix* to fill the wound with disorganized *granulation tissue*, largely composed of collagen (primarily collagen type III), fibronectin, and hyaluronan.[32] While various matrix metalloproteinases (MMPs) are released to breakdown damaged tissue throughout this phase, new tissue synthesis generally exceeds tissue degradation.

Additionally, new blood vessels form through a process called *angiogenesis* to support the newly developing granulation tissue with nutrients necessary for growth, including oxygen and energy, as well as removal of hazardous waste products.[33] Inflammatory macrophages secrete a number of angiogenic factors to attract vascular endothelial cells and stimulate vessel formation. Mural cells or pericytes are recruited to newly formed capillaries to become smooth muscle cells that line the blood vessels and help to stabilize them for the formation of new endothelial cell lined vessels. Proliferation and ECM repair continues for approximately 6 weeks.

In dermal healing, re-epithelialization occurs as keratinocytes migrate from the edges of the granulation tissue and then proliferate to form a barrier. Wound contraction also plays an important role in dermal healing, as dermal fibroblasts differentiate into myofibroblasts, adhere to the wound edges through desmosomes, and contract, similarly to smooth muscle cells, reducing the wound size.

1.1.5 REMODELING

The final remodeling stage of healing may last for weeks to months. Cells *remodel* the provisional granulation tissue matrix to remove disorganized scar tissue and maintain functional tissue. Cells slow their ECM production, eventually reaching a balance of tissue synthesis and degradation by MMPs. In collagenous tissues, collagen is remodeled from disorganized collagen III rich tissue into more organized collagen I fibrils during this time. Remodeling is important for prevention of scar tissue formation, as excessive fibrous tissue production results in scarring. Remodeling results in a mechanically stronger and more organized tissue that closely resembles the pre-injury tissue. Remodeling may last for several months.

1.1.6 ROLE OF MATRIX METALLOPROTEINASES (MMPs) AND TISSUE INHIBITORS OF MATRIX METALLOPROTEINASES (TIMPs) IN TISSUE REGENERATION AND MAINTENANCE

Matrix metalloproteinases (MMPs) and their inhibitors, called tissue inhibitors of metalloproteinases (TIMPs), play critical roles in tissue regeneration and remodeling. All cell types in the body express varying amounts of MMP to remove damaged ECM and replace it with newly synthesized tissue, and MMP activity is carefully controlled by TIMPs.[34, 35] Additionally, MMPs are also naturally produced by cells to facilitate normal proliferation, migration, differentiation, cell signaling, and angiogenesis.[34, 35] A balance of MMP and TIMP activity, in combination with new tissue synthesis, is necessary for tissue regeneration and healthy tissue maintenance. During the Proliferation stage of healing, MMPs are responsible for breaking down damaged tissue, while new tissue synthesis generally exceeds tissue degradation, resulting in a bulk increase in tissue deposition. During the Remodeling stage, MMP activity continues to break down disorganized scar tissue and replace it with organized matrix, reaching a balance of tissue synthesis and degradation by MMPs. This remodeling continues throughout the life of the tissue as matrix is degraded and replaced to maintain the health and structure of the tissue. As discussed in the following section, however, overexpression of MMPs can result in tissue destruction and prevent healing, as observed in some chronic wounds. In contrast, underexpression of MMPs may result in tissue scarring during healing, indicating that a delicate balance of MMP and TIMP expression is critical to achieve truly regenerative healing and preferred outcomes.

1.1.7 RESOLUTION OF HEALING AND RESTORATION OF TISSUE HOMEOSTASIS

Following the remodeling stage of healing, the healing response gradually diminishes, and the tissue returns to normal homeostasis. The cell-rich, highly vascular granulation tissue is replaced with organized ECM, and cell numbers decrease in the tissue as a portion of cells undergo apoptosis.[36] Simultaneously, many of the small blood vessels that formed to support the granulation tissue dissociate, and the remaining vessels mature to form fully functional vascular networks.[32, 37] The inflammation response also diminishes as immune cells undergo apoptosis, migrate out of the tissues, or their activity is suppressed by immunomodulatory signals.[37] Cellular debris is finally phagocytosed and removed from the tissue by macrophages to prevent the persistence of inflammation. As the tissue enters homeostasis, the tissue matures into a highly organized, matrix-rich environment in which cells continually maintain and remodel the ECM and supporting vasculature.

1.2 OBSTACLES TO HEALING

Despite the body's ability to heal naturally, a number of impediments may impair one of the three phases of healing and often result in scarring or loss of function in injured or diseased tissue. For example, small wounds will often regenerate tissue with no signs of damage, while wounds that are larger in size, become infected, or are in patients in poor health may result in scarring that is both aesthetically distinct and functionally less pliable than healthy tissue. Remodeling of deep injuries, such as severe burns, is complex, especially when damaged dermal layers are unable to provide cells for repair. Similarly, complex neural injuries or diseases that require extensive neural regeneration present unique challenges in tissue remodeling and repair. Some common obstacles to healing include severe tissue damage, poor vascularization, and impaired regulation of inflammation.

When *severe tissue damage* occurs as part of a traumatic injury, resident cells are often unable to fully regenerate the damaged tissue. The body's natural response is to immediately close off the wound to prevent blood loss, infection, and ultimately death; therefore, such wounds tend to fill with disorganized fibrous scar tissue. Even though these large open wounds do eventually close, the scar tissue that fills the wound does not fully replicate the properties or appearance of the original tissue. Additionally, because tissue regeneration is a complex process requiring highly regulated molecular signals, the lack of an appropriate scaffold for tissue repair, vascular insufficiency, and the absence of coordinated cellular signals in severe injuries limit the ability of cells to repair the original tissue. As a result, excessive or disorganized collagen production to fill the wound may lead to fibrosis and scarring.

Poor blood supply to tissues may occur in patients having diabetes, for example, and result in ischemic (or having deficient blood supply) tissue, particularly in the extremities, that lacks access to nutrients, oxygenation, and reparative cells. This most often occurs in the lower extremities which endure the largest forces in supporting the body's weight while also being most distant from the heart, which is the source of blood flow. Wounds may occur in poorly vascularized tissues and rather than undergoing normal tissue repair the wounds may worsen, forming a chronic wound. As a result of poor blood supply, the wounds may not receive the necessary signals to heal properly. Poor vascularization also coincides with a *low availability of circulatory stem cells* from the bloodstream, and reparative cells, including immune cells and stem cells, may be unable to populate the wound to stimulate repair or may enter a hostile environment that is not conducive to the repair process. Such deficiencies often occur as a result of diabetes, and may result in the formation of diabetic foot ulcers (DFUs), as shown in Figure 4. Similarly, naturally avascular tissues like tendon, ligament, and cartilage have a low ability for healing partially due to limited blood supply.

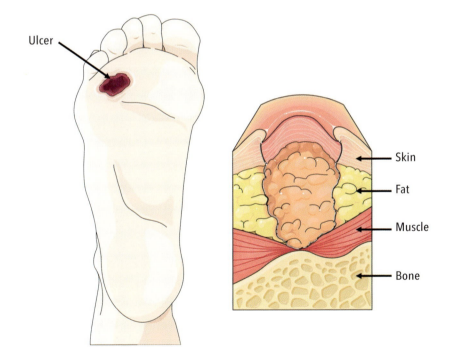

Figure 4. Diabetic foot ulcer. Diabetic foot ulcers may expose layers of skin, fat, muscle, and/or bone. [b]

[b] Figure from http://www.servier.com/Powerpoint-image-bank (Servier Medical Art By Servier, Diabetes, Creative Commons Attribution 3.0 Unported)

In addition, *disease states*, such as diabetes, often may result in unhealthy tissues and impaired responses. Effects from disease itself may impair the healing response through abnormalities in the tissue architecture, the cellular response, or the signaling environment. *Medications* used to treat the ailments (such as immunosuppressive drugs, chemotherapy drugs, etc.) add another facet that may disrupt healing responses through their unintended consequences on the body and cellular environments.

An *impaired inflammatory response* may also result from an improper balance of immunomodulatory cues. As a result, the healing process can be impaired and the chronically inflamed tissues can be overwhelmed with high levels of MMPs and proteases, excessive levels of destructive reactive oxygen species, or uncontrolled levels of infection. It has been reported that 28% of chronic wounds have high levels of MMPs.[38] In chronic wounds, sustained inflammation and often infection plague the wound, thus preventing the resolution of inflammation and inhibiting the ability to activate the additional signals necessary to progress through the proliferation and remodeling stages of healing, as shown in Figure 5.

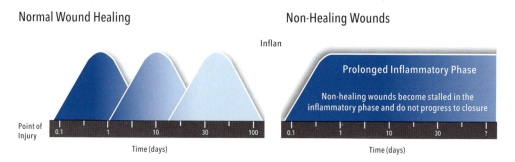

Figure 5. Prolonged inflammation in chronic wounds prevents progression through the normal wound healing process.

In chronic wounds, activated neutrophils have been shown to persist over time. These neutrophils continue to produce enzymes, including MMP-8, elastase, and gelatinase, that degrade the tissue matrix. The activity of these MMPs is out of balance with TIMPs and α2-macroglobulin. Macrophages are also present, and secrete MMPs including an increased expression of MMP-1, -2, -3, -9, -13 and reactive oxygen species, creating a highly oxidative environment. Reactive oxygen species (ROS) are free radicals derived from oxygen containing byproducts. ROS are highly reactive molecules that can cause damage to cells and ECM. Although these harsh environments occur naturally to clear bacteria and necrotic tissue from the wounds, in chronic wounds the signals required to end inflammation are impaired. Inflammatory cytokines, including TNF-α, IL-1, and IL-6, dominate the wound environment, while repair cytokines that promote proliferation and ECM production, such as PDGF and TGF-β, are reduced in the wound exudates.[39]

The causes of these wounds are unclear, though they appear to involve both local and systemic stimuli. The effects of hyperglycemia in diabetes, increased hydrostatic pressure, tissue hypoxia, nonphysiological pH, presence of bacterial components and foreign bodies, and fragments of necrotic tissue perpetuate the inflammatory response and, as a result, the persistent tissue damage in chronic wounds.

The keys to resolution of inflammation are currently not well understood. Application of anti-inflammatory factors alone has not resulted in the development of effective therapies to promote healing. Therefore, regulation of a balance of pro- and anti-inflammatory regulatory molecules may be required to reset the wound trajectory from one of chronic inflammation to one of acute healing to progress through the natural healing process.

1.3 THERAPIES TO PROMOTE HEALING

The goal of regenerative therapies is to modulate these stages of healing, including modulation of inflammation, cell migration and proliferation, and tissue remodeling, in order to promote the body's natural ability to repair. Interventions to promote and improve healing are being developed to overcome these obstacles. Nonbiological therapies such as hyperbaric oxygen, low-level laser therapy, and negative pressure therapy may contribute to healing through various molecular pathways, including modulation of local and circulating immunomodulatory molecules[40] and may provide a potential role in various combination therapies; however, these therapies are outside of the scope of this Primer.

The use of tissue grafts, including an in depth discussion of MiMedx PURION® Processed amniotic membrane allografts, is addressed in Chapter 2 of this Primer.

AMNIOTIC MEMBRANE ALLOGRAFTS FOR TISSUE REPAIR

2.1 TISSUE GRAFTS FOR REPAIR

Tissue grafts have been used for a number of regenerative medicine applications. These grafts use naturally created tissues to restore function and promote repair in damaged tissues. *Autografts* are tissues harvested from one area of the body and implanted into the *same* patient to replace an injured tissue. The major limitations of autografts are the limited supply of donor tissue available and the morbidity and pain associated with the donor site for the patient. Healthy tissue intended for use in the repair has to be surgically removed from the afflicted patient through a "secondary" surgery while attempting to minimize the creation of an additional wound that will limit function or result in donor site morbidity; therefore, with a number of injuries and diseases, harvesting autograft tissue is not an option.

Allografts, however, are harvested from a tissue donor and implanted into a *different* patient. Allograft tissue is removed from either a living donor or a cadaver and preserved until use. Tissues are most commonly stored frozen or cryopreserved; however, some nonviable tissues can also be dehydrated and stored at room temperature or ambient conditions until use. Unlike autografts, these allografts do not require secondary surgery in the patient for tissue harvest; however, use of allografts may include additional risk of disease transmission. Therefore allografts require review of thorough patient history records and infectious disease testing prior to implantation. Allografts also may carry the risk of an unfavorable immunogenic response from the recipient if the recipient's body recognizes and mounts an immunological response against the foreign human leukocyte antigen (HLA) antigens in the donor tissue. Although some tissues may be harvested from immunologically privileged sites, for non-immunologically privileged tissues, organ matching and/or taking immunosuppressants may be required.

Xenografts are grafts that are transplanted between different species, such as grafts harvested from *animal tissues* for implantation into human patients. Though xenografts do not have the same availability concerns as autografts and allografts, xenografts have to undergo aggressive processing to remove immunogenic animal products from the tissue. This includes thorough decellularization to remove cellular components prior to use, leaving only an extracellular matrix tissue scaffold with limited biological activity.

Each tissue graft type requires different processing and storage techniques. Some of the common tissue processing techniques are described below.

2.1.1 DECELLULARIZATION

Tissue processing generally requires cleansing to remove potentially hazardous byproducts from the tissue. The most extreme processing involves complete decellularization to remove all cellular components from the graft (examples: Alliqua BioMedical BIOVANCE®, Smith and Nephew Oasis®, TEI Biosciences PriMatrix®, DePuy Synthes DermaMatrix™). Decellularization is generally performed in order to remove immunogenic cellular components and prevent immune rejection by the recipient. Decellularization washes out cellular byproducts including bioactive regulatory factors, leaving only a mechanically intact but biologically inert extracellular matrix scaffold which may be repopulated with the patient's own cells. This is similar to collagen-based scaffolds, which can be produced from animal-derived collagens and manufactured into scaffolds that, while not naturally derived, also lack cells and bioactive growth factors (example: Integra® Wound Matrix). Decellularization is a requirement in xenograft tissues (examples: Smith and Nephew Oasis, TEI Biosciences PriMatrix), due to the immunogenic potential of the animal cells in these nonhuman tissues. Decellularization is also required in non-immunologically privileged tissues such as human dermis, which contains human HLA antigens and would be at risk of immune rejection.

2.1.2 CRYOPRESERVATION

The most common method to preserve tissue grafts and prevent degradation is through cryopreservation or freezing (examples: Osiris® Grafix®, Amniox® NEOX®). Freezing tissue can prevent degradation by reducing enzymatic and chemical activity in the tissues and inhibiting the growth of microorganisms. The major limitation of cryopreservation is that tissues are typically frozen, stored, and thawed under controlled temperature conditions and in cryoprotectants, such as dimethylsulfoxide (DMSO) and glycerol that are added to prevent ice crystal formation within the tissues and preserve tissue integrity.

As water freezes, ice crystals may form in the tissue and these crystals can destroy the cellular membranes, thus killing cells and disrupting tissue matrix. Thus, cryopreserved tissues generally require cryoprotectants to prevent ice crystal formation; however, such cryoprotectants can also be cytotoxic at high concentrations or extended exposure times and must be thoroughly rinsed from the product after thawing and prior to application on patients. Cryopreservation is also typically limited to small or thin tissues, as larger tissues are difficult to control cooling temperature throughout, resulting in ice formation in thick or larger tissues. Cryopreserved grafts are also difficult to transport and store, often requiring flash freezing in liquid nitrogen, shipping on dry ice, and storage in large, temperature controlled freezers, most often at -80°C or below. Additional challenges may be encountered during the thawing process, where if the grafts are not closely monitored and controlled, cells may experience stress that results in cell death.

2.1.3 DEHYDRATION

An alternative to cryopreservation is tissue dehydration (examples: MiMedx EpiFix® and AmnioFix®, BioD® DryFlex®, Derma Sciences AmnioExcel®, Alliqua BioMedical BIOVANCE, Applied Biologics™ XWRAP®, DePuy Synthes DermaMatrix, TEI Biosciences PriMatrix, Smith and Nephew Oasis). Tissue can be dehydrated under heat, open air, or freeze drying (lyophilization). Dehydration preserves tissue without the need for freezers, dry ice, or liquid nitrogen, which are required for storage of cryopreserved grafts. By removing residual moisture from the tissue, the tissue is preserved by reducing activity of soluble chemical reactions and water-dependent enzymatic activity and inhibiting the viability of microorganisms in the low moisture environment. Certain methods of dehydration have been shown to retain equivalent or superior biological activity to cryopreservation, with the added benefit of producing product that may be shipped and stored at room temperature or ambient conditions and which is easier to handle.

By removing water from the tissue, dehydration may alter the tissue's microstructure by causing the matrix to become more compact in the absence of water. Dehydrated tissues are typically mechanically stronger and easier to handle than wet tissues. However, the tissue matrix proteins remain preserved, and in the wound, the dehydrated tissue is rehydrated, returning the tissue to its original state. Once hydrated, the tissue matrix is bioactive and can be degraded by MMPs and remodeled by host cells, becoming incorporated into host tissues and eventually being replaced with native, host tissue.

2.1.4 LIVE CELL THERAPIES

Due to their regenerative potential, delivery of autologous or allogeneic mesenchymal stem cells (MSCs) has attracted attention as a potential therapeutic approach for repair and regeneration of damaged tissue. The rationale behind delivering living cells to a wound is that they may substitute for, or augment the activity of, the patient's own cells, which are presumed to be lacking in number or competence. However, poor engraftment and survival of the cells at the site of injury are major limiting factors preventing the efficacy of live cell therapies in the clinic. It has been widely reported that the number or percentage of delivered stem cells that actually engraft, or take up residence, in a wound is extremely low, and even the small number of cells that do engraft disappear from the wound very quickly after implantation, either by dispersion or death.[41-43] Therefore, while live stem cell therapies may demonstrate viability in optimized *in vitro* conditions, viable cells are often no longer present after several days following implantation into the body, and any influence of the delivered cells on the wounds may be short lived.

Similar live somatic cell therapies, including bioengineered cell-based grafts for dermal tissue healing (examples: Organogenesis Apligraf® and Dermagraft®), have seen similar insufficiencies of poor cell viability and engraftment.[44-46] Similar to implanted MSCs, the fibroblasts and keratinocytes present in the grafts, while viable during *in vitro* culture and at the time of implantation, are likely to rapidly undergo apoptosis in the harsh wound environments and do not persist in the wounds.[44-46] In addition, these complex cell-based grafts remain expensive, wasteful if the wound size is smaller than the one large graft sheet size available, and may be difficult to use in the clinic due to all the preparation steps required prior to use. Additionally a comparative clinical trial demonstrated that PURION Processed dHACM was more effective healing diabetic wounds than a leading bioengineered live cell graft, suggesting that live cells may not be necessary for improved healing clinically.[47]

The poor viability of transplanted cells is often amplified by the harsh wound environments into which the cells are implanted. In necrotic or chronically inflamed environments, implanted cells rapidly undergo apoptosis and cell lysis, releasing their apoptotic contents and signals into the wound. Therefore, these live cell therapies (example: Osiris Grafix, Organogenesis Apligraf and Dermagraft) may in fact be *here today and gone tomorrow.* Poor engraftment and survival of implanted cells remain significant obstacles which must be overcome before live cells can be routinely used to effectively promote healing and regeneration.[41-43]

2.2 AMNIOTIC MEMBRANE ALLOGRAFTS

Biological tissues from a variety of sources have been used to treat wounds. Human skin autografts and allografts have been employed for burns and chronic wounds, as well as bone and tendon/ligament autografts and allografts for orthopedic repair.[48-50] A number of animal-derived xenograft tissues including porcine and bovine skin (example: TEI Biosciences PriMatrix), urinary bladder, and small intestinal submucosa (SIS; example: Smith and Nephew Oasis) have been developed and marketed for surgical repair, wound care, and burn care.[51-53] Non-immunologically privileged allografts (harvested from a human tissue donor) and xenografts (harvested from animal tissues) typically require decellularization to remove immunoreactive cellular components, leaving a biologically inert acellular extracellular matrix scaffold with limited amounts of bioactive factors, which may lead to a less effective healing response.

In 2006, Surgical Biologics, now a wholly owned subsidiary of MiMedx, developed the PURION Process for cleansing and dehydration of amniotic membrane allografts. Randall Spencer, co-founder of Surgical Biologics and Vice President of Clinical Innovation at MiMedx, was instrumental in leading the development of the PURION Process, and over the years, this process was improved, perfected, and eventually protected through nearly 20 issued patents since 2012.[54-70] Human amniotic membranes in the form of minimally processed fresh, frozen, or dehydrated tissue allografts have increased in popularity as barrier membranes to promote healing of dermal, ophthalmic, and surgical wounds, partly due to their immunologically privileged properties. Treatment of wounds with amniotic tissues provides a biological barrier for the wound, while *modulating inflammation, reducing scar tissue formation, and enhancing soft tissue healing.*[71, 72]

Recently a number of amniotic-derived grafts have been introduced with limited scientific and clinical studies to support their efficacy (examples: Osiris Grafix, Amniox NEOX 100, BioD DryFlex, Derma Sciences AmnioExcel, Alliqua BioMedical BIOVANCE, Applied Biologics XWRAP). While it is possible that further critical studies may be eventually conducted on these newer grafts, MiMedx has published over 22 peer-reviewed scientific and clinical articles since 2012 documenting the clinical efficacy and cellular mechanisms behind PURION Processed dHACM, setting a standard for scientific and clinically-based evidence.[47, 73-94]

Documented in this text are numerous studies demonstrating that amniotic membrane allografts are not created equal, nor do they have the same clinical responses.

Human amniotic membrane is derived from the inner and outer layers of the amniotic sac and is comprised of two distinct but conjoined membranes – amnion and chorion. The amnion faces the fetus and the chorion faces the uterus. The membranes consist of organized collagen-rich extracellular matrix, viable cells, and regulatory proteins and signaling molecules. The amnion and chorion contain no blood vessels and have no direct blood supply.[95] Required nutrients are supplied to the amniotic membranes directly by diffusion out of the amniotic fluid or from the underlining decidua.[72] Likewise, the membranes also secrete substances both into the amniotic fluid and toward the uterus, influencing both amniotic fluid homeostasis and maternal cellular physiology, respectively.[96]

As depicted in Figure 6, amnion is composed of five distinct layers, including the epithelium, basement membrane, compact layer, fibroblast layer, and intermediate or spongy layer. The epithelium, the layer closest to the developing fetus, consists of a single layer of epithelial cells uniformly arranged on the basement membrane.[72] The basement membrane is a thin layer composed of collagens III and IV and noncollagenous glycoproteins laminin, nidogen and fibronectin.[97] The compact layer is a dense layer almost totally devoid of cells and forms the main fibrous structure of the amnion.[95, 97] Interstitial collagens I and III form bundles in the compact layer that maintain the mechanical integrity of the membrane, while collagens V and VI form filamentous connections to the basement membrane.[97] The fibroblast layer is the thickest layer of the amnion and consists of fibroblasts embedded in a loose collagen network with islands of noncollageneous glycoproteins.[95, 97] The outermost spongy layer forms the interface between the amnion and chorion, composed of a nonfibrillar meshwork of collagen III and an abundant content of proteoglycans and glycoproteins.[72, 97]

The chorion layer is three to four times thicker than the amnion.[98, 99] Chorion is composed of a reticular layer, basement membrane, and trophoblast layer which is adhered to the maternal decidua on the placental disc, but not in the amniotic sac.[97] The reticular layer contacts the spongy layer of the amnion and forms a majority of chorion's thickness.[100] The reticular network is composed of collagens I, III, IV, V, and VI.[97] The basement

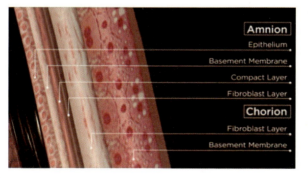

Figure 6. Layers of the amniotic membrane including the amnion and chorion.

membrane anchors the trophoblasts to the reticular layer with collagen IV, fibronectin, and laminin.[97, 100] The trophoblast layer is the deepest layer, consisting of 2 to 10 layers of trophoblasts which contact with the decidua on the surface of the placenta.[100]

Placental tissues are known to play important roles in nutrient transport to the fetus, removal of waste products, and exchange of oxygen and carbon dioxide through the mother's blood supply, as well as preventing exposure of the fetus to harmful bacteria and viruses.[96] Research continues to further investigate the many roles of the placenta in regulating pregnancy, including its importance in fetal development.[96, 101]

During pregnancy, the amniotic membrane in particular acts as a naturally derived, biologically active, and mechanically robust barrier between the mother and child. The amniotic membrane holds the developing fetus and amniotic fluid, so this thin membrane must possess the *structural integrity* to support the pregnancy through term.[97] It must also continue to grow to accommodate the increasing volume of the conceptus, and therefore it is a metabolically active tissue which continually remodels and grows. Remodeling of the tissue is governed by *growth factors, cytokines, chemokines, extracellular matrix*, and *related regulatory factors* produced by the endogenous cells in the amniotic membrane. This tissue must grow and expand without scar tissue formation to successfully carry the growing child.

In addition to physically encasing the amniotic fluid and developing fetus, amniotic membranes play an integral biological role in fetal development and progression of pregnancy; therefore, amniotic membrane grafts harbor significant biological activity, including a number of developmental cytokines that play important roles is tissue formation. As a biological barrier between the mother and child, amniotic tissues are naturally designed to contain low levels of HLA-A, -B, and -C antigens and beta 2-microglobulin and are therefore considered *immunologically privileged* tissues for allograft transplantation.[88] For these reasons, amniotic membrane tissue has been shown to be a biologically derived tissue that acts as a natural barrier to promote healing in chronic and surgical wounds.

While other placental materials such as *umbilical cord* and *amniotic fluid* are currently under investigation as candidate allograft tissues, there are currently *little to no published randomized controlled clinical trials* to support their use in healing and tissue regeneration. Umbilical cord and amniotic fluid are distinct tissues from the amniotic membrane. Umbilical cord is composed of Wharton's jelly surrounding the umbilical vein and two umbilical arteries. Wharton's jelly is a gelatinous substance made largely from hyaluronan and a diffuse collagen extracellular matrix, as well as low cellularity of fibroblasts.[102]

As a liquid, amniotic fluid is predominantly composed of water that is derived from maternal plasma and contains carbohydrates, proteins, lipids, electrolytes, and urea, along with low cellularity of a heterogeneous population of naturally-derived cells.[103]

2.2.1 PLACENTA DONATION PROCESS

MiMedx placental tissues are supplied through donation programs across the United States. Industry standards include that the donation of tissue only come from mothers delivering full-term babies via scheduled Caesarean section. There are medical conditions that can disqualify a donor mother, including active cancer and infectious diseases.

Prospective donor mothers typically learn of placenta donation through their Obstetrician's office. Prior to their scheduled Caesarean section surgery date, they are informed of the program, allowed to ask questions and receive informative responses, and must sign an Informed Consent, consistent with guidelines issued by the American Association of Tissue Banks, to allow donation of their placental tissues. Each prospective donor mother must also fill out a medical/social questionnaire and have a simple blood test. This test is performed at the same time as the admittance blood draw, and therefore requires no additional needle sticks. Serology performed from that blood sample includes testing for human immunodeficiency virus (HIV), human T-lymphotropic virus (HTLV), syphilis, cytomegalovirus (CMV), Hepatitis B, and Hepatitis C.

After delivery, MiMedx has its own recovery technicians who will work with the delivery team to recover the delivered placenta. Nothing additional is required of the mother. Once the tissue has been recovered, it is immediately transported to a MiMedx processing facility. The placenta is placed in quarantine storage until the serology reports confirm acceptable results.

2.2.2 ADVANTAGES OF THE MIMEDX PURION® PROCESS

The goal of tissue processing is to cleanse the tissue of hazardous material, while retaining the natural properties of the original tissue; therefore, MiMedx formulated the PURION Process specifically for amniotic membrane tissue in 2006. The proprietary PURION Process acts to gently cleanse the amniotic tissue, while preserving the structural integrity and biochemical activity of amniotic membrane. While amniotic cells are rendered nonviable, these cells remain intact, including cellular and pericellular components that are essential for biological activity. The gentle PURION Process preserves the natural structure of the cells, thereby maintaining the bioactive factors associated with the cells *in vivo*. Retention of bioactive factors is thought to be critical for the clinical efficacy of the tissue allograft in wound repair and tissue regeneration. Dehydration preserves the grafts at ambient temperature for up to 5 years, while allowing for easy handling during implantation. ***Therefore, by preserving the native amniotic membrane in a dehydrated, easy-to-use tissue matrix, the PURION Process provides a distinct advantage over amniotic membrane allografts processed using less effective alternative methods.***

The PURION Process is used to produce *dehydrated human amnion/chorion membrane* (dHACM) allografts (e.g., EpiFix and AmnioFix). In PURION Processed dHACM grafts, chorion is dissected from the amniotic sac and not from the placenta or chorionic plate; therefore, the chorion tissue is non-maternally derived and presents a low risk of eliciting an immune response. The chorion tissue is approximately three to four times greater thickness over amnion alone; therefore, when combined with the gentle cleansing PURION Process, dHACM grafts generally contain twenty times greater growth factors and cytokines than competitive single layer and amnion only grafts[104] (examples: Osiris Grafix, Amniox NEOX 100, BioD DryFlex, DermaSciences AmnioExcel, Alliqua BioMedical BIOVANCE, Applied Biologics XWRAP, AlloSource® Allowrap® DS).

While there are several different types of amnion/chorion laminate grafts in clinical use, PURION Processed dHACM has still been shown to contain higher quantities of growth factors and cytokines than many of these products.[104, 105] Analysis of PURION Processed dHACM suggests that the PURION Process is a gentle cleansing process that retains a high proportion of the biologically active factors that are naturally present in amniotic tissues. One can theorize that other products with lower growth factor and cytokine retention likely utilize a harsher cleansing process that washes bioactive material out of the grafts and greatly reduces the cytokine content and natural composition of the tissues. This indicates that *not all amnion/chorion bilayer grafts are processed equally.*

The primary objective of the PURION Process is to ensure a safe allograft product for the patient, while preserving the biological activity of the native amniotic membrane. As a result, PURION Processed dHACM does contain low levels of MMPs and traditional "pro-inflammatory" cytokines that are naturally present in amniotic tissue.[107, 108] These molecules are produced physiologically by amniotic cells and play critical roles in tissue development in native amniotic membrane tissues;[109,110] therefore, they should be viewed as regulatory molecules for tissue regeneration, remodeling, and healing, rather than misleadingly labeled as "destructive" or "inflammatory" molecules. Only when expressed in excess are these molecules harmful and counterproductive to healing. All bioactive proteins within the amniotic membrane are at normal physiological levels; therefore, PURION Processed dHACM only retains physiological levels of cytokines, as they are naturally present in native amniotic tissues to support fetal development.[107, 108]

The chorion tissue used in PURION Processed dHACM grafts is *sourced from the amniotic sac alone* as shown in Figure 7, and not from the placenta or chorionic plate. Therefore, this chorionic tissue is not maternally derived and is immunologically privileged, suggesting that dHACM possesses a low potential for eliciting an immune response. All dHACM grafts were shown to contain low levels of HLA antigens similar to native amnion tissues.[111] In further support of the safety of MiMedx dHACM grafts in clinical use, over 450,000 PURION Processed allografts have been distributed since 2006 with zero FDA reportable adverse reactions.

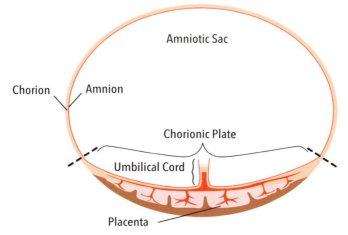

Figure 7. Cross-section of placental tissues. During Caesarean section procedures and after the baby has been delivered, the placental tissues including the amniotic sac, umbilical cord, and the placenta are removed from the mother. Chorion tissue is sourced only from the amniotic sac (indicated by the hashed lines) and not the chorionic plate, which contains maternal tissue.

In addition to being processed using aseptic methods, PURION Processed dHACM grafts are also *terminally sterilized* by gamma ray or electron beam irradiation to further reduce the risk of disease transmission. Though high levels of radiation may potentially crosslink or denature proteins within tissues, an examination of dHACM grafts before and after terminal sterilization demonstrated that sterilization by irradiation did not affect the cytokine content of the grafts, growth factor elution out of the grafts, histological appearance, or their ability to promote fibroblast proliferation, suggesting that sterilization does not alter the bioactivity of the dHACM grafts while ensuring maximal safety to the patients.[112]

As a result, MiMedx PURION Processed dHACM allografts are specifically processed to retain the native bioactivity of the amniotic membrane while preserving the grafts in a dehydrated tissue matrix, in order to maximize efficacy and promote tissue healing. Despite the number of competitive amniotic membrane allografts currently on the market that are attempting to replicate this technology, *not all amniotic membrane allografts are equal, and the PURION Process provides a distinct advantage over other amniotic membrane allografts that are processed using alternative techniques.*[76, 105, 106] MiMedx PURION Processed dHACM allografts have been optimized to:

- Retain the native bioactivity of amniotic membrane tissue
- Provide a thick tissue graft with more growth factors, cytokines, and tissue matrix than thinner single layer grafts
- Have a low risk of immunological rejection
- Reduce the risk of disease transmission with terminal sterilization
- Allow storage at ambient conditions for up to 5 years
- Be easy to use and handle

CHAPTER 3

RELEVANT CELL TYPES FOR TISSUE REGENERATION

As mentioned previously, cells are the biological building blocks of tissue. They maintain the function of the tissue by synthesizing proteins or metabolizing waste. Single cells communicate with one another and respond to stimuli in their surrounding environments through soluble signaling molecules, including cytokines, growth factors, hormones, steroids, enzymes, and other chemicals. The body is composed of a vast number of cell types. Each is unique to specific tissues and possesses unique functions in the body. A number of relevant cell types are described below, including resident cell types, vascular cells, stem cells, and immune cells.

3.1 RESIDENT TISSUE CELLS

Each tissue contains specific cell types that reside in the tissue and are responsible for the biological function, maintenance, and renewal of the tissue. Upon injury, these cells release coordinated signals to stimulate a healing response. During the healing process, resident cells are responsible for aiding and providing the regenerative cells to replace the damaged tissue with new, healthy tissue. These resident cells include connective tissue cells, as well as, epithelial, endothelial, nerve, and immune cells. Connective tissue cells, also known as mesenchymal cells, are a family of cells grouped together based upon the similarities they share in origin, character, and interchangeability, including fibroblasts, cartilage cells, bone cells, fat cells, and smooth muscle cells. Despite the variety of cell types comprising the connective tissue cell family, they share the role of secretion of fibrillar and non-fibrillar extracellular matrix and general architectural framework. The mesenchymal stromal or stem cells (MSCs) that reside in every tissue and organ have high replicative and differentiation potential. They play a critical role in support and repair, and the adaptability of their differentiated character is an important feature of tissue responses to many types of damage.[113] The various cells residing in skin, tendon and ligament, muscle, heart, bone, cartilage, and fat tissues are discussed in the following sections.

3.1.1 SKIN CELLS: FIBROBLASTS AND KERATINOCYTES

3.1.1.1 DERMAL FIBROBLASTS

Fibroblast and fibrocyte is terminology that has been historically used to describe two states of the same mesenchymal cell type. A suffix of -blast is typically used to denote the activated state of metabolism and replicative potential for a cell; whereas, -cyte is the less active state involved in maintenance of the surrounding tissue. However, rarely are the two states differentiated from each other, and the cells are more commonly called fibroblasts.

Morphologically, fibroblasts in tissues and in culture show an elongated, branched cytoplasm, surrounding an elliptical, speckled nucleus which contains two or more nucleoli. Metabolically active, replicative fibroblasts are recognized by their larger size, more prominent nucleus, and increased rough endoplasmic reticulum. Inactive or "poised for action" tissue fibrocytes are notably smaller, spindle shaped and contain less rough endoplasmic reticulum.

Fibroblasts are the most common connective tissue cell present in the body where their primary role is maintaining the structural integrity of connective tissue. They are dispersed through the dense tissue where they produce a collagen subunit, tropocollagen, which is used to assemble larger collagenous aggregates. They also produce glycosaminoglycans, elastic fibers, reticular fibers, and glycoproteins to create an extracellular matrix (ECM). Fibroblasts, collagen, and ECM provide the framework for connective tissue, otherwise referred to as the "stroma" in animal and human tissues.

Human dermal fibroblasts (HDFs) are cells that reside within the dermis layer of skin where they are responsible for uniting the dermis and epidermis through the generation and maintenance of the connective tissue and secretion of molecules important to maintain homeostasis. The fibroblasts produce an extracellular matrix (ECM) rich in laminin and fibronectin which allows the epithelial cells of the epidermis to affix to the matrix, thereby allowing the epidermal cells to effectively join together to form the top layer of the skin. They also produce a variety of growth, differentiation, and protective factors.

HDFs are responsive to both chemical and physical stimulation. Proliferation can be induced in these cells in the presence of various enzymes and growth factors, including fibroblast growth factor (FGF). Also, when the dermis layer is disrupted due to injury, HDFs can proliferate and migrate to the site of damage where they deposit new ECM rich in type I and type III collagen. The fibroblasts at the site of injury are also able to respond to the injury as a cue to begin expressing α-smooth muscle actin and differentiate into myofibroblasts. This allows the fibroblasts to actively migrate to a damaged site, and then to slowly contract and seal the skin after an injury to prevent infection.

3.1.1.2 KERATINOCYTES

Keratinocytes are dermal epithelial cells that make up a majority of the epidermis, which is the outermost layer of skin, as shown in Figure 8. Keratinocytes primarily form a barrier between the body and the external environment, including protection against bacteria, ultraviolet radiation, heat loss, and water loss. Keratinocytes form from dividing progenitor cells in the basal layer or stratum basale of the epidermis, which is the deepest layer. As the cells differentiate, they reside in the stratum spinosum layer, have decreased replicative potential, and produce keratin, which acts as the structural component of the stratum corneum, or tough outer layer of skin. Eventually, keratinocytes will undergo terminal differentiation, in which they die, forming a nonviable component of the stratum corneum.

Keratinocytes also play an important role in tissue homeostasis, including regulation of inflammation at the skin barrier to battle infections. Keratinocytes produce inflammatory cytokines, adhesion molecules, and chemotactic factors, including TNF-α, IFN-γ, TGF-β, IL-1, and IL-10 that activate microvascular endothelial cells and immune cells in the dermis and epidermis and stimulate cutaneous inflammation.[114]

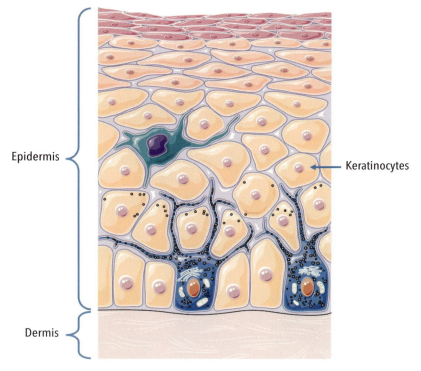

Figure 8. Keratinocytes in the epidermis.[c]

3.1.2 TENDON AND LIGAMENT CELLS: FIBROBLASTS

Similar to dermal fibroblasts, tendon and ligament tissue contains fibroblast cells that are interspersed between collagen fiber bundles and are responsible for synthesizing and maintaining the ECM of the tissue. Tendon and ligament fibroblasts, which are also referred to as tenocytes in tendon, are critical for the preservation of tendon/ligament mechanical strength, and also participate in remodeling the tissue during healing. In response to injury, fibroblasts attract reparative cells through chemotactic signals, release endogenous growth factors, and help elicit innate and adaptive immune responses. Tendon and ligament fibroblasts communicate with each other to respond and adapt to conditions of increased mechanical load with changes in gene expression and ECM synthesis. Tendons and ligaments, however, are poorly vascularized tissues that lack blood vessels, and many tendons and ligaments do not heal or regenerate without surgical intervention.

3.1.3 SKELETAL MUSCLE CELLS: MYOBLASTS AND MYOCYTES

Muscle cells include skeletal myoblasts and myocytes, smooth muscle cells, and cardiomyocytes. *Skeletal muscle* includes all of the striated muscles that voluntarily control bodily movement. Skeletal muscle attaches to bone through tendons, and contracts to impart forces on the skeleton. *Smooth muscle* includes involuntary non-striated muscle which includes muscles in the walls of blood vessels, lymphatic vessels, urinary bladder, gastrointestinal tract, respiratory tract, erector pili of skin, ciliary muscle, and iris of the eye, uterus, and male and female reproductive tracts. Smooth muscle cells contract in response to various involuntary stimuli, including chemical or mechanical signals, to control critical bodily functions. *Cardiac muscle* includes involuntary striated muscle of the heart. Cardiac muscle propels blood through the heart chambers, lungs, and circulatory vessels.

Myoblasts are progenitor cells that divide and differentiate into myocytes. Myocytes are muscle cells that contract to induce movement. Contraction stimuli trigger an action potential which causes the release of intracellular Ca^{2+}. Thick myosin filaments, thin actin filaments, and elastic titin filaments work together in myocytes to produce cellular contraction, as depicted in Figure 9. Myosin undergoes a conformation change that pulls on the actin filaments and causes cellular contraction. Synchronized contraction of individual myocytes causes the entire muscle to contract simultaneously.

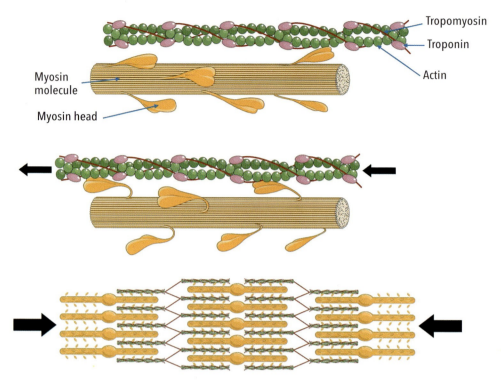

Myosin molecule

Myosin head

Tropomyosin

Troponin

Actin

Figure 9. Muscle sarcomere including myosin and actin. Myosin undergoes a conformation change that pulls on the actin filaments and causes cellular contraction.[d]

3.1.4 HEART CELLS: CARDIAC FIBROBLASTS AND CARDIOMYOCYTES

Human Cardiac Fibroblasts (HCFs) are the most prevalent cell type in the heart, comprising 60-70% of all cells. They play a central role in the maintenance of the ECM in the normal heart and the synthesis of growth factors and cytokines. Under pathological conditions, cardiac fibroblasts are involved in scar formation following myocardial infarction, cardiac fibrosis, and cardiac hypertrophy.

As mentioned previously, cardiac muscle includes involuntary striated muscle of the heart. Cardiomyocytes are the muscle cells that contract to propel blood through the heart chambers, lungs, and circulatory vessels.

[d] Figure from http://www.servier.com/Powerpoint-image-bank (Servier Medical Art By Servier, Muscles, Creative Commons Attribution 3.0 Unported)

3.1.5 BONE CELLS: OSTEOBLASTS, OSTEOCLASTS, AND OSTEOCYTES

Bone is a very dense, specialized form of connective tissue. Bone matrix is comprised of type I collagen fibrils and solid particles of hydroxyapatite. This composition allows bone to resist pulling and compression forces necessary for its function. The extracellular matrix is fairly rigid; however, about 15% of the weight is occupied by the living cells in the ECM. The primary role of these cells is remodeling bone matrix. Osteoblasts are bone forming cells that can divide, produce dense, crosslinked Type I collagen, and mineralize bone. Osteoclasts are bone degrading cells that can divide and work in balance with osteoblasts to break down and remodel bone matrix as a normal homeostatic process. As osteoblasts are trapped by the mineralized matrix they secrete, they become differentiated osteocytes which are responsible for maintaining the matrix tissue. Osteocytes do not proliferate, but they regulate bone matrix remodeling through mechanosensory mechanisms and signal transduction to control activity of osteoblasts and osteoclasts.

3.1.6 CARTILAGE CELLS: CHONDROCYTES

Chondrocytes are the cells that are responsible for synthesizing, degrading, and maintaining cartilage tissue. Cartilage is flexible connective tissue that lines the surface of joints and composes structural tissue in the rib cage, ear, nose, bronchial tubes, and intervertebral discs. Cartilage is relatively rigid with strong compressive strength, yet also flexible enough for cushioning during load bearing due to high water content in the tissue. Chondrocytes maintain the complex ECM network of cartilage through normal ECM turnover. Chondrocytes have been shown to alter their expression to respond to mechanical forces during loading. However, cartilage is an avascular tissue that lacks blood vessels and access to progenitor cells, resulting in a poor capacity for healing and regeneration without surgical intervention.

3.1.7 FAT CELLS: ADIPOCYTES

Human fat cells or adipocytes are derived from fibroblast-like cells during development and in some instances, pathological circumstances. Fibroblast-like precursor cells are converted to mature fat cells by the accumulation and coalescence of lipid droplets in the form of triglycerides and cholesterol. The role of an adipocyte is to store reserves of energy and to generate energy to meet the demands of the body, including temperature regulation. Though fat is often viewed negatively because an overabundance of fat is commonly associated with poor health, adipose tissue plays important roles in regular tissue maintenance throughout the body, including storage of energy, cushioning from impact, and insulation of heat. As discussed in Section 3.3.2, adipose tissue also acts as a stem cell niche for a population of adipose-derived stem cells, which are part of the stromal vascular fraction of fat tissue.

3.2 VASCULAR CELLS

Blood vessels transport blood and nutrients throughout the body. As shown in Figure 10, blood vessels are composed of a thick wall of connective tissue on the exterior, layers of smooth muscle cells in the middle layer, and a thin layer of endothelial cells lining the interior surface of the vessel. These cell layers control transportation of cells and nutrient in and out of the circulation to the surrounding tissues. The connective tissue also provides structural strength and elasticity and the smooth muscle controls vasoconstriction and vasodilation to alter blood flow in response to stimuli.

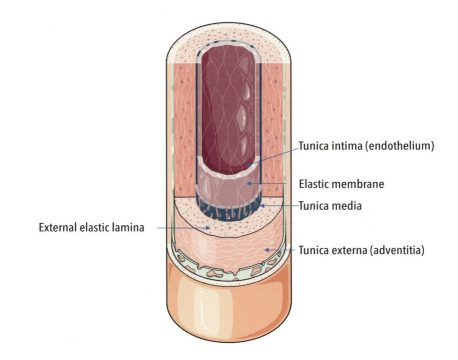

Figure 10. Blood vessels are composed of connective tissue on the exterior, smooth muscle in the middle, and endothelium on the interior.[e]

---

[e] Figure from http://www.servier.com/Powerpoint-image-bank (Servier Medical Art By Servier, Muscles, Creative Commons Attribution 3.0 Unported)

3.2.1 VASCULAR ENDOTHELIAL CELLS

The vascular endothelium acts as a selective barrier between the lumen and surrounding tissue in order to control the flow of materials in and out of the bloodstream. Endothelial cells are highly involved in sprouting angiogenesis, which involves the formation of capillaries by activated endothelial cells branching out from an existing capillary. There is a surrounding matrix that the endothelial cells will use to form a cordlike structure. Angiogenesis involves many factors such as basic fibroblast growth factor (bFGF) and vascular endothelial growth factor (VEGF) which are involved in endothelial cell growth and differentiation. Transforming growth factor-β (TGF-β) and angiogenin are two factors that inhibit endothelial cell proliferation and promote differentiation, both necessary for the healthy development of blood vessels and capillaries.[115-117]

3.2.2 VASCULAR SMOOTH MUSCLE CELLS

The intima layer of a blood vessel is made up of a thick layer of smooth muscle cells. These cells are responsible for the contraction and relaxation of blood vessels, which enables the vessels to have a fitting blood pressure based on blood flow. During vessel remodeling, smooth muscle cells produce extracellular matrix components and increase their proliferation and migration. Platelet-derived growth factor (PDGF) is one factor responsible for the migration of smooth muscle cells. The process begins with an endothelial cell tube forming and then the migration of smooth muscle progenitor cells. With the two cell types working together, along with many more cell types and proteins, normal blood vessel formation is a coordinated effort with multiple players.[118, 119]

3.3 ADULT STEM CELLS

Adult stem cells are multipotent stem and progenitor cells that are present in adult (non-embryonic) tissues, and can differentiate to form different cells and tissues throughout the body. Adult stem cells play critical roles in normal bodily function and maintenance and also respond to injury to promote healing.

3.3.1 MESENCHYMAL STEM CELLS

Mesenchymal stem cells (MSCs) are adult stem cells that are found traditionally in the bone marrow, and have also been identified as components of bone marrow, umbilical cord, and fat tissues. Found throughout the body, MSCs are now thought to be comprised of dividing and quiescent cells capable of self-renewal, and it has been proposed that MSCs may be pericytes residing in association with blood vessels where they can be rapidly

31

mobilized in response to tissue injury.[120] MSCs are self-renewing and multipotent. *Self-renewing* means that these cells are capable of dividing to replicate themselves. They are stimulated to divide and actively migrate to sites of injury where they participate at multiple levels in the repair process. *Multipotent* means that these adult stem cells can differentiate into more than one specialized cell type, with limitations. This differs from *pluripotent* (embryonic) stem cells which do not have limitations and can form any of the three embryonic germ layer cell types, including endoderm, mesoderm, and ectoderm. As depicted in Figure 11, MSCs can undergo a mesengenic process whereby they can specifically differentiate into fat, cartilage, bone, tendons, muscle, dermal tissue, and potentially other cell types, such neural and endothelial cells.[121] In addition, under the right conditions MSCs may transdifferentiate into epithelial cells.[122] With these collective properties, MSCs are essential and valuable in tissue repair and renewal. Because adult MSCs are not immunologically rejected acutely, and they are not ethically controversial due to their post-birth derivation, they are a primary focus for therapeutic applications and research. Surface markers for MSCs include CD44, CD73, CD90, CD105, CD117, and stem cell antigen 1 (Sca-1), but MSCs from different organs and those cultured *in vitro* display a variety of phenotypic differences that are just beginning to be understood and defined.

Mesenchymal Stem Cell

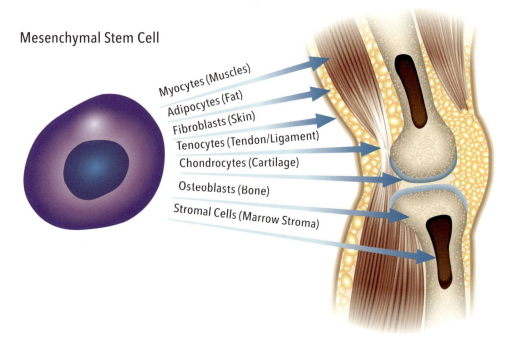

Myocytes (Muscles)
Adipocytes (Fat)
Fibroblasts (Skin)
Tenocytes (Tendon/Ligament)
Chondrocytes (Cartilage)
Osteoblasts (Bone)
Stromal Cells (Marrow Stroma)

Figure 11. MSCs are adult stem cells that can differentiate into a number of mesenchymal lineages. Mesenchymal stem cells are multipotent and possess the ability to proliferate and commit to different cell types based on the environmental conditions.

MSCs are found in all tissues and are essential for general tissue maintenance and also injury repair. They produce and respond to a variety of signaling molecules. *Cytokine* is a general term used for all signaling molecules produced by cells for specific biological functions, including growth stimulation, while *chemokines* are specific cytokines that function by attracting cells to sites of infection/inflammation. For example, IL-8 is a type of chemokine produced by cells as a "chemo-attractant" that calls in reparative cells, including MSCs, which migrate and home to the injury site, where they also release cytokines into the repair microenvironment. Once signaled, MSCs circulate via peripheral blood to the tissue where they are needed to assist with repair.[121] One of the essential chemokines in the selective migration and tissue retention of MSCs is SDF-1α (stromal cell derived factor-1α).[123, 124]

Specific MSC differentiation pathways can be induced by external factors such as hormones, growth factors, cytokines, and extracellular matrix (ECM) proteins, which regulate gene expression inside the cell.[125] Essentially, a combination of environmental factors and molecular cues dictate how the stem cell should behave.

One of the greatest initiators of differentiation is a process called paracrine signaling. *Paracrine signaling* is a cell to cell communication in which signals secreted by one cell impact the behavior of nearby cells. Not only are MSCs impacted by these secreted factors, they themselves are also powerful regulators of surrounding cells by their own paracrine activity. Just a few of the many cytokines secreted by MSCs are fibroblast growth factor (FGF) and epithelial growth factor (EGF), which cause an increase in local fibroblast and epithelial proliferation, respectively. MSCs also secrete vascular endothelial growth factor (VEGF), angiopoetin-1 (Ang-1), and platelet-derived growth factor (PDGF) which enhance blood vessel formation.[126] In addition, the paracrine signals from MSCs play a role in the modulation of inflammation.[127]

3.3.2 ADIPOSE DERIVED STEM CELLS

As mentioned previously, MSCs can also be derived from the stromal vascular fraction (SVF) of fat tissue, in which case they are referred to as adipose derived stem cells (ADSCs). ADSCs share similar cell surface markers and genetic profiles to MSCs originating in bone marrow.[128] Direct comparisons between human ADSCs, bone marrow MSCs, and other MSCs have demonstrated that many of the proteins they express are nearly identical when cultured under similar conditions,[129] but there are still a number of differences between MSCs when cultured in various microenvironments and *in situ*.[130] Fat tissue is a ready source from both autologous and allogeneic donors, and millions more ADSCs can be derived from the initial SVF, when compared to bone marrow or other MSC sources. Therefore, ADSCs are being explored as a therapeutic option for various clinical indications, due to the less invasive nature by which they are obtained for autologous use (i.e., liposuction), their surrounding proximity to a wound, and their robust ability to divide and be expanded *in vitro*.

3.3.3 HEMATOPOIETIC STEM CELLS

Hematopoietic stem cells (HSCs) are adult stems cells that differentiate into myeloid and lymphoid blood cell lineages, as shown in Figure 12. Myeloid cells include monocytes and macrophages, neutrophils, basophils, eosinophils, erythrocytes or red blood cells, megakaryocytes or platelets, and dendritic cells, while lymphoid cells include T cells, B cells, and natural killer cells. HSCs are primarily found in the bone marrow niche, but they can be recruited into the circulation by chemokines and therefore are also present in peripheral blood.[131] As with other stem cells, they are self-renewing and multipotent. Unlike MSCs, however, HSCs are non-adherent cells, meaning that they are cultured while suspended in liquid media and do not adhere to tissue culture-treated plastic. They also have different growth requirements than MSCs. Cell surface markers for HSCs include CD45, CD133, and CD105, and negative for standard lineage markers of HSC differentiation.

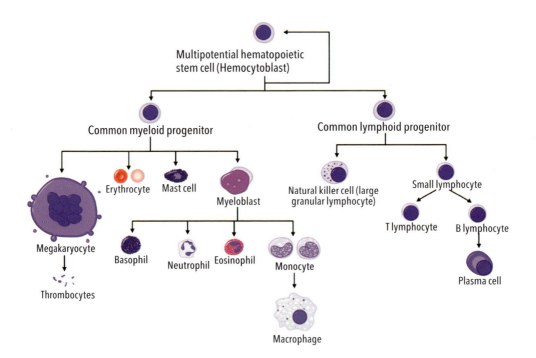

Figure 12. HSCs are adult stem cells that can differentiate into all of the blood cell lineages.[f]

---

[f] Figure from http://commons.wikimedia.org/wiki/File:Hematopoiesis_simple.svg (from original http://commons.wikimedia.org/wiki/File:Hematopoiesis_(human)_diagram.png by A. Rad, Creative Commons Attribution-Share Alike 3.0 Unported)

These surface markers are used for identification of HSCs from other cell types; however, due to interspecies variation, common HSC markers also differ slightly across humans and mice, which are commonly used experimentally in HSC studies. For example, human HSCs are positive for CD34, CD59, CD90/Thy1 markers, while in mice, HSCs are positive for CD38, Sca-1, and c-Kit (which is a receptor for stem cell factor).

Bone marrow transplants are routinely used as treatment for blood cancers and disorders, such as leukemia, lymphoma, and multiple myeloma. In this treatment regimen, cancerous cells are killed using high dose chemotherapy and/or radiation therapy in the host, such that the stem cells in the blood and bone marrow are depleted. The impaired HSCs are then replaced with healthy allogeneic HSCs that are collected from either bone marrow or from peripheral blood of a healthy donor, which is matched with the recipient to prevent or reduce the risk of rejection and/or graft-versus-host reactions.[131]

3.4 IMMUNE CELLS

As previously discussed in Section 1.1.2 on Inflammation, white blood cells or leukocytes are cells of the immune system which are responsible for protecting the body against infectious disease and foreign invaders. The immune system includes innate and adaptive immune responses. The innate immune system acts as the first line of defense to rapidly and nonspecifically respond to foreign pathogens. The adaptive or acquired immune system, however, responds to pathogens to create a long-term immunological memory. As a result, the adaptive immune system can initiate a heightened response to subsequent exposures to the same pathogen and provide a protective immunity. Leukocytes can be classified as granulocytes, monocytes/macrophages, and lymphocytes. Granulocytes include neutrophils, eosinophils, basophils and mast cells, while lymphocytes include T cells, B cells, and natural killer cells.

3.4.1 NEUTROPHILS

Neutrophils are granulocytes that make up 60-70% of all circulating leukocytes. Neutrophils primarily fight infection through the process of *phagocytosis*, where a cell engulfs and digests pathogens and tissue debris in response to microorganisms and necrotic tissue.[2] Neutrophils are the first responders to microbial infection, and they engulf and eat bacteria and release *free radicals (also referred to as "reactive oxygen species" or "ROS")* to kill infectious agents and suppress infection.[1] Neutrophils also release pro- and anti-inflammatory immunomodulatory *cytokines*, including TNF-α, IL-1α, IL-1β, IL-ra, IL-3, IL-12, IFN-γ, TGF-β, GCSF, MCSF, and GM-CSF. In addition, neutrophils secrete *chemokines* like IL-8, MIP-1α, MIP-1β, and MCP-1, which attract monocytes/macrophages into a wound, and *angiogenic growth factors* like VEGF and HGF, which are important for promotion of the formation of new blood vessels.[3] Collectively these molecules stimulate tissue regeneration by host cells, as well as having downstream effects on monocytes, granulocytes, and lymphocytes. After engulfing pathogens, neutrophils die and are removed by the body.

3.4.2 EOSINOPHILS

Eosinophils are granulocytes that respond to allergic stimuli, parasitic infections, and disease. They are relatively rare in blood, and are primarily found in mucous membranes of the respiratory, digestive, and lower urinary tracts. In response to infection, eosinophils degranulate, releasing the contents of their granules which are toxic to pathogens. They also release reactive oxygen species, enzymes, angiogenic growth factors such as TGF-β, VEGF, and PDGF, and immunomodulatory cytokines such as IL-1, IL-2, IL-4, IL-5, IL-6, IL-8, IL-13, and TNF-α.

3.4.3 BASOPHILS AND MAST CELLS

Basophils and *mast cells* are granulocytes that contain granules rich in histamine and heparin, and respond to parasitic infections, wounds, and allergic stimuli. Basophils and mast cells release histamine and heparin, altering blood coagulation and acute inflammation. Basophils and mast cells are also an important source of IL-4 secretion, an important immunomodulatory cytokine that is involved in regulation of the immune system.[132] Though similar in function, basophils circulate in the bloodstream, while mast cells reside in connective tissues. Basophils, however, can be recruited out of circulation into tissue in response to stimuli.

3.4.4 MONOCYTES AND MACROPHAGES

Monocytes are recruited to damaged tissues, in response to chemokines including RANTES, MIP-1α/β, I-309, and MCP-1, which are released by platelets and neutrophils.[7] After leaving the bloodstream and entering the damaged tissue, monocytes differentiate into macrophages. These macrophages play roles in innate and adaptive immunity. They are primarily responsible for engulfing foreign bodies and damaged tissue, similar to neutrophils, but macrophages also play an important role in releasing signals which stimulate blood vessel formation and tissue formation. Macrophages are known to secrete TGF-α, TGF-β, PDGF, IGF-I, TNF-α, IL-1, and IL-6.[2] These signals recruit new fibroblasts and lymphocytes to the wound and promote granulation tissue and angiogenesis. Macrophages also produce *reactive oxygen species* which kill bacteria within the wounds, and are involved in tissue remodeling through expression of MMPs

36

and TIMPs.[2] Unlike neutrophils, macrophages can replace their lysosomal contents and have a longer lifespan and presence in the wounds.

Activated macrophages have been shown to differentiate into two distinct phenotypes, which are referred to as the "classically activated" M1 and "alternatively activated" M2 macrophages.[8-10] These phenotypes work in concert to balance inflammation within the wounds. "Classically activated" M1 macrophages engulf foreign pathogens, and generally promote an increase in inflammation including release of IL-1β, IL-6, IL-12, and TNF-α, as well as secretion of chemokines like IL-8, IP-10/CXCL10, MIP-1α, MIP-1β, and RANTES.[8-10, 13] M1 macrophages also produce MMPs-1, -2, -7, -9, -12 which enzymatically degrade ECM.[14, 15]

"Alternatively activated" M2 macrophages, on the other hand, are typically associated with reduction of inflammation and promotion of tissue repair.[8-10] M2 macrophages decrease overall inflammation and encourage tissue repair through release of anti-inflammatory factors such as IL-1Ra, IL-10, and TGF-β and chemokines such as MDC/CCL22, PARC/CCL18, and TARC/CCL17.[18-23] M2 macrophages also assist the repair process by secreting fibrogenic and angiogenic growth factors, such as PDGF, IGF, TGF-β, bFGF, TGF-α, and VEGF.[24, 25] These molecules secreted by M2 macrophages contribute toward the resolution of inflammation and promotion of wound repair.

Both of these macrophage phenotypes work together to regulate a reparative immune response, not alone in isolation; therefore, the balance of M1 and M2 activity is an important marker of the healing response and the relative contributions of the two phenotypes.[29]

3.4.5 LYMPHOCYTES

Lymphocytes include T cells, B cells, and natural killer cells. T lymphocytes recognize "non-self" antigens, and mount a response to eliminate foreign pathogens. T cells can be classified as cytotoxic, helper, and suppressor T cells. *Cytotoxic T cells*, which carry the surface marker CD8, bind major histocompatibility complex I (MHC I) expressed on the surface of virus-infected cells and kill them. Cytotoxic T cells are generally believed to downregulate repair processes. *Helper T cells*, which are positive for CD4, are activated by binding MHC II on antigen presenting cells (such as macrophages and dendritic cells), where they activate and regulate T and B cells.[2] Similar to M1/M2 polarization of macrophages, helper T cells also differentiate into Th1 and Th2 cells. Th1 cells activate macrophages and heighten immune response against intracellular bacteria, in response to IL-2 and IFN-γ. Th2 cells activate eosinophils, basophils, and mast cells and heighten response against extracellular parasites, in response to IL-4. Helper T cells are considered to promote tissue regeneration. This balance of helper and cytotoxic T cells is required to regulate fibrous tissue growth and promote repair through angiogenic and fibrogenic factors. *γδ T cells* are a unique population of T cells that do not require MHC presentation for cytotoxic destruction. γδ T cells may have an important role in recognition of lipid antigens.

B lymphocytes are responsible for producing antibodies that recognize, bind, and block pathogens and mark them for removal and destruction. B cell receptors bind an antigen, which is internalized by the cell, and fragments of the antigen are presented on the cell surface in a complex with MHC class II receptors. Helper T cells bind the MHC II/antigen complex and promote B cell activation into plasma or memory B cells. *Plasma B cells* rapidly secrete antibodies of different immunoglobulin (Ig) classes (mainly IgM, IgG, and IgA) specific to that antigen into the bloodstream, which mark the pathogens for destruction by phagocytes. *Memory B cells* express surface immunoglobulins specific to the antigens and survive for longer periods of time, facilitating a rapid response in case of secondary exposure to that antigen. Memory B cells are part of the previously described "adaptive" immune response, providing longer term immunity against pathogens.

Natural killer (NK) cells are cytotoxic lymphocytes that kill virally infected cells of the body, similar to cytotoxic T cells. Unlike cytotoxic T cells, however, NK cells respond rapidly as part of innate immunity and can recognize stressed cells in the absence of antibodies or MHC. NK cells release cytotoxic granules containing perforin and granzymes which perforate and kill the infected cells.

CHAPTER 4

STRUCTURAL PROTEINS AND EXTRACELLULAR MATRIX IN TISSUE REGENERATION AND HEALING

Tissues are made of cells embedded or otherwise attached to extracellular matrices. The extracellular matrix (ECM) serves two major functions. It provides structural support for the cells and mechanical properties for the tissue, while also playing important roles in regulating cellular activity.[133] The relative proportion of ECM varies according to the function of the tissue. Tissues and organs such as liver, pancreas, and spleen contain mostly cells that are held together by a sparse ECM framework. In tissues like tendons and ligaments where the mechanical properties are central to the tissue's function, the ECM is vastly predominant and the few embedded cells play mainly growth, maintenance, and reparative roles.

The key elements comprising extracellular matrices are the structural proteins, collagens, and elastin, specialized proteins like laminin and fibronectin, and proteoglycans.[133] Collagen forms fiber arrays which are responsible for strength and stiffness of the ECM, but also provide binding domains for the resident cells and templates for organizing the non-collagen ECM components.[134] Interspersed within the collagen fiber networks are supramolecular aggregates of ECM macromolecules, which themselves are highly organized. Specialized proteins are part of some tissues, like the protein elastin super polymers found in lung and aorta and the glycosaminoglycan hyaluronic acid. The relative contents of these ECM macromolecules likewise vary according to tissue function.

4.1 COLLAGEN

Over 25 distinct types of collagen have been identified in human tissues. Types I, II, and III are the major fiber forming collagens and they account for most of the collagen in the body.[134, 135] Type IV collagen forms network arrays and has limited distribution as the structural non-fibrillar foundation for epithelial tissues.[136] Types

V and VI collagen are associated with Type I collagen in most interstitial tissues and are prevalent in placenta.[137] Type VII collagen forms anchoring fibrils that connect the epidermis to the dermis in skin.[138] Type VIII collagen is associated with a variety of endothelial cells.[139] Type IX collagen is localized in cartilage where it is bound to Type II collagen fibrils.[140] Type X collagen is found in mineralizing cartilage where it participates in accretion of minerals.[141] Type XI collagen forms small fibrils in articular cartilage.[141] A brief description of the major collagen types that are important for tissue regeneration follows.

Table I. Collagen Types I – XI, structure and tissue distribution.

COLLAGEN TYPE	STRUCTURE	TISSUE DISTRIBUTION
Type I	Fibrils and fibers	Most abundant collagen of the human body. It is found in tendons, skin, artery walls, cornea, the endomysium surrounding muscle fibers, fibrocartilage, and the organic part of bones and teeth.[134] It is present in scar tissue, the end product when tissue heals by repair.[143]
Type II	Small fibrils	Hyaline cartilage, makes up 50% of all cartilage protein. Vitreous humour of the eye.[134]
Type III	Small fibrils	Produced quickly by young fibroblasts before the tougher type I collagen is synthesized. Reticular fiber. Often associated with Type I collagen. Also found in artery walls, skin, intestines and the uterus. This is the collagen of granulation tissue.[143]
Type IV	Non-fibrillar networks	Basal lamina; foundation for epithelial cells. Also serves as part of the filtration system in capillaries and the glomeruli of nephron in the kidney.[136]
Type V	Small fibers	Most interstitial tissue, associated with Type I, associated with placenta.[137]
Type VI	Microfibrils, forms beaded filaments	Most interstitial tissue, associated with Type I.[137]
Type VII	Anchoring fibrils	Forms anchoring fibrils in dermoepidermal junctions.[138]
Type VIII	Non-fibrillar short chain collagen, forms hexagonal lattices	A variety of endothelial cells.[139]
Type IX	Attached to type II collagen fibrils	Fibril associated (FACIT) collagen, cartilage, associated with Type II and XI fibrils.[142]
Type X	Non-fibrillar short chain collagen, forms hexagonal lattices	Hypertrophic and mineralizing cartilage.[141]
Type XI	Small fibers	Cartilage.[142]

Type I collagen forms large aggregates of linearly arrayed collagen molecules. The fundamental unit of all Type I collagen fibrous systems is the fibril. Collagen molecules align end to end in a ¼ to ¾ staggered overlap with neighboring molecules resulting in the 67 nanometer banded pattern observed with the electron microscope (Figure 13).[144] This aggregation or polymerization occurs through physicochemical interactions. The exact alignment of the collagen molecules within fibrils is crucial for fibril stability and mechanics.[145] This is true for all fibrillar collagens. As the collagen molecules aggregate into fibrils, covalent cross-linking proceeds through specific amino acids, typically lysine. Formation of these intermolecular covalent cross-links is mediated by an enzyme, lysyl oxidase, that forms the reactive lysine species that then go on to form adducts with specific amino acids with neighboring collagen molecules.[134] Proper cross-link formation relies on proper alignment of the molecules within the fibril. Proper fibril mechanics relies on proper intermolecular cross-linking.

Collagen fibrils associate in linear arrays to form fibers (Figure 13). Type I collagen fibers function primarily in tension.

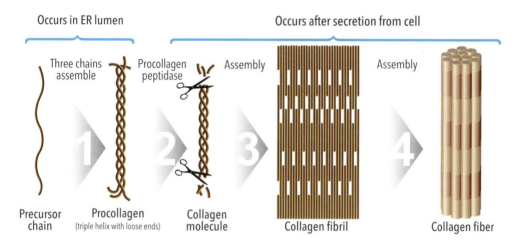

Figure 13. Assembly of collagen molecules into fibrils and fibers.

The organization of the Type I collagen fibers is tissue specific. In tendon, all fibers run parallel with the longitudinal axis of the tendon,[146] as shown in Figure 14. They function to transmit the mechanical force of muscle to bone. They must be strong enough to withstand the muscular force, and stiff enough to not stretch as the muscle shortens. The strength and stiffness of tendon tissue is derived entirely from the collagen fiber system, which accounts for over 90% of the tissue substance.[146, 147]

Tendon Structure

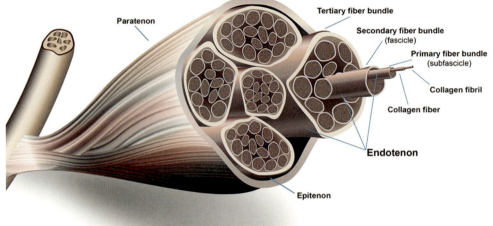

Figure 14. The hierarchical structure of Type I collagen in tendon.

Ligaments are similarly composed of linear arrays of Type I collagen fibers. Ligaments connect the articulating bones in synovial joints, and therefore are strong and stiff like tendons. However, since ligaments undergo three dimensional deformations (as opposed to purely linear loads in tendon), the fiber architecture, while still linear in overall direction, is arranged in twisted arrays.[147] In that way, different fascicular elements come under tension at various angles of extension and flexion.

In skin, the Type I collagen fibers are arranged in a network array with no preferred orientation.[148] This allows the skin to deform in any direction. As skin is deformed, the collagen network becomes aligned in the direction of load.[148] Once the fibers are aligned, deformation is no longer possible. When the force is removed, the fibers return to their normal network organization, and the skin returns to its normal shape.

Muscle contains an extensive Type I collagen network which binds muscle fibers into a cohesive unit (Figure 15).[149] The smallest dimensional element is the endomysium surrounding muscle fibers. These units are then bound together by the perimysium forming a fascicle. The muscle fascicles are held together by the epimysium.[150] Force transmission in muscle relies on this collagen fiber architecture.

The organic phase of bone is predominantly Type I collagen fibers. The collagen functions as the nucleation site for the accretion of bone mineral. Calcium based minerals in the form of hydroxyapatite intercalate within collagen fibrils.[151] Mineralization of the collagen fibrillar system is responsible for bone strength and stiffness. The microstructure of bone is depicted in Figure 16.

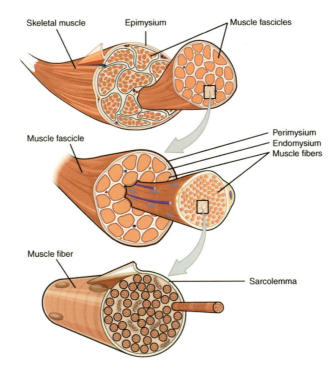

Figure 15. Muscle structure showing the intrinsic Type I collagen fiber system: muscle fibers are bound together by endomysium and fascicles are bound together by perimysium. The entire structure is held together by epimysium. All of these tissues are composed primarily of Type I collagen fibers.[g]

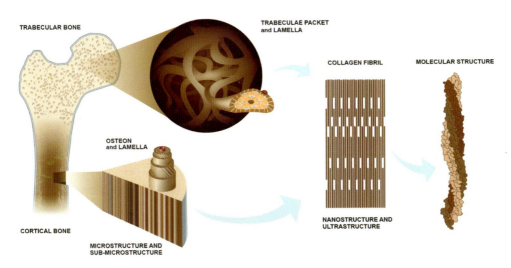

Figure 16. The structure of bone and mineralization of Type I collagen fibrils.

[g] Figure from http://commons.wikimedia.org/wiki/File:1007_Muscle_Fibes_(large).jpg (Anatomy & Physiology, Connexions Web site. http://cnx.org/content/col11496/1.6/, Jun 19, 2013., Creative Commons Attribution 3.0 Unported)

Type II collagen is found primarily in articular cartilage capping the bones in synovial joints and in hyaline cartilages such as nose, ear, and trachea. Type II collagen forms thin fibrils in a network array and accounts for approximately 50% of the ECM (Figure 17).[134, 142] The function of the Type II network is to constrain the high concentration of proteoglycan aggregates (described below).[152]

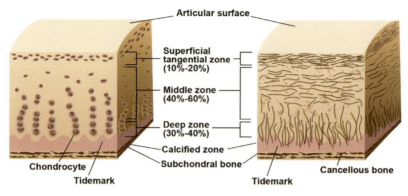

Figure 17. Structure of cartilage showing the Type II collagen fibrillar system. Left cross-section shows chondrocytes embedded in the ECM. Right cross-section shows the orientation of collagen fibrils in the ECM.[142]

Type III collagen is a fibrillar collagen similar in structure to Type I collagen. It forms thin fibers and is sometimes found incorporated into Type I collagen fibers.[143] Its function is not clearly understood, but it appears early in the development of ECMs. It is enriched in fetal and neonatal tissues and is almost always associated with Type I collagen fibers.[153] It is present in relatively high amounts in arteries, skin, intestine and uterus. Type III collagen is expressed in relatively high amounts in regenerating tissues.

Type IV collagen is the major structural element in basal lamina and basement membranes and is restricted to tissues with epithelial elements where it forms sheets of dense fibrillar networks.[136] It forms the foundation on which epithelial cells are attached. It some tissues it functions as a filtration membrane.[136] Tissues rich in Type IV collagen include epidermis, kidney, and amniotic membranes. The presence of collagen IV in human amnion and chorion membranes is shown in Figure 18.

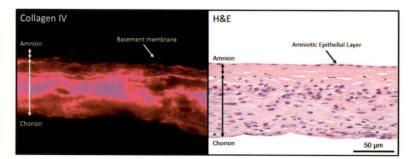

Figure 18. Collagen Type IV staining on the left and hematoxylin and eosin (H&E) staining on the right of dehydrated human amnion/chorion membrane.

44

Type V collagen is a fibrillar collagen that is present in most collagenous tissues. It is often associated with Type I collagen fibrils and, in some tissues, is incorporated into Type I collagen fibrils.[154] It is enriched in basement membranes where it can function as a substrate for cell binding.[154]

4.2 ELASTIN

Elastin is a large protein polymer that has reversible elastic properties. It is made up of highly cross-linked elastin molecules,[155] as depicted in Figure 19. It provides the tissue with the ability to repeatedly undergo large deformations. It is localized to tissues that must reversibly change shape, like lung, aorta, and cardiovascular tissues.[155] In skin, it is responsible for the dermis's elasticity. Elastic fibers are also found in the chorion of amniotic membrane.

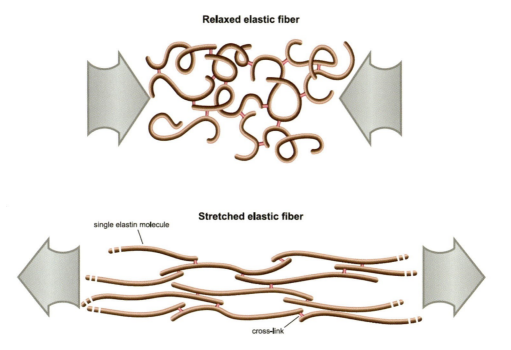

Figure 19. Schematic representation of cross-linked elastin fiber networks which undergo reversible deformation.

4.3 LAMININ

Laminins are large, multifunctional, structural proteins in the extracellular matrix and are specifically concentrated in basal lamina of basement membranes where they are associated with Type IV collagen.[156] The laminin molecule is comprised of three distinct subunits that assemble into a cross-like structure (Figure 20). It can associate with a variety of ECM macromolecules via specific binding domains, including collagen and proteoglycan binding domains.[156] It contains binding domains for cells via the integrins on cell membranes.[156] Thus, laminins are an integral part of the ECM scaffolding and its intimate connections with the resident cells.

Laminin Molecular Structure

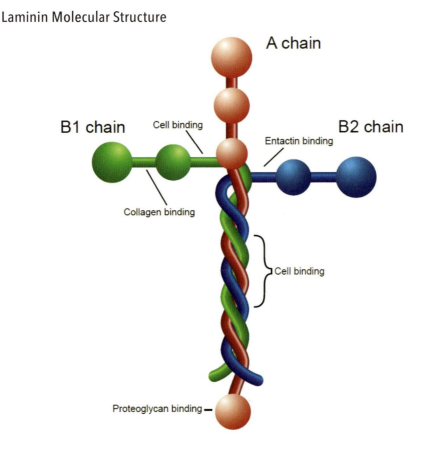

Figure 20. Model of laminin molecule. The laminin structure is composed of the three peptides that form the cross shaped conformation including functional binding domains for collagen, proteoglycans, and cells.

4.4 FIBRONECTIN

Fibronectin is a large glycoprotein of the ECM where it functions as a substrate for cell binding. It contains specific amino acid sequences which the cell membrane-spanning integrins bind strongly,[157] as shown in Figure 21. Therefore, it can serve as a facilitating substrate for cell adhesion, growth, proliferation, migration, and differentiation. It also contains binding domains for ECM macromolecules, specifically collagen and heparan sulfate proteoglycans.[157] As such, it functions as the nexus of the ECM-cell interface.

Fibronectin Interaction

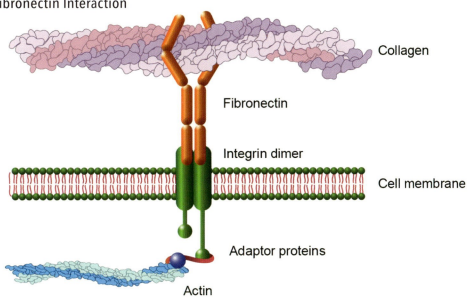

Collagen

Fibronectin

Integrin dimer

Cell membrane

Adaptor proteins

Actin

Figure 21. Illustration of the structure of fibronectin and its associations with fibrillar collagen and the cell surface integrin binding domains in the extracellular space.

4.5 MATRIX METALLOPROTEINASES (MMPs) AND TISSUE INHIBITORS OF MATRIX METALLOPROTEINASES (TIMPs)

Matrix metalloproteinases (MMPs) are zinc protease enzymes that degrade extracellular proteins. There are currently 24 different MMPs, and most are directed towards degrading ECM structural proteins like collagens and proteoglycans. Additional MMP substrates include cytokines, chemokines, growth factors, binding proteins, cell/cell adhesion molecules, and other proteinases. Some common MMPs are shown in Table II, including two of the six membrane-type MMPs (MT-MMPs). Each MMP has a specific target in the ECM, is produced to affect a particular process, and is produced by certain types of cells.[158] They are important because many of the structural proteins of the ECM, especially the fibrillar networks, are not degraded by most enzymes. The MMPs are specifically produced to remodel the ECM and associated cellular and structural components. MMPs are integrally involved in embryonic development, normal differentiation, morphogenesis, tissue growth, cell migration, angiogenesis, and reproduction.[159] They are also involved in diseases where inappropriate and sometimes chronic ECM remodeling is a consequence of the pathology.

Table II. Common matrix metalloproteinases (MMPs) involved in tissue remodeling that are secreted into the ECM.

MMP	NAME	DESCRIPTION
MMP 1	collagenase	Cleaves triple helical collagen molecules in fibers producing two fragments that can then be degraded by gelatinases.[160]
MMP 2	gelatinase	Degrades collagens IV and V in basement membranes, and the gelatin produced following collagenase cleavage.[160, 161]
MMP 3	stromelysin	Cleaves many ECM proteins but is not able to degrade fibrillar collagen.[160]
MMP 8	neutrophil collagenase	Degrades fibrillar collagens.[160]
MMP 9	gelatinase	Degrades collagens IV and V in basement membranes, and the gelatin produced following collagenase cleavage.[160, 161]
MMP 10	stromelysin	Cleaves many ECM proteins but is not able to degrade fibrillar collagen.[160]
MMP 12	elastase	Degrades elastin, fibronectin, Type IV collagen.[161]
MMP 13	collagenase 3	Cleaves fibrillar collagen.[160]
MMP 14	protease	MT-MMP; found in high concentrations in placental tissues, involved in MSC and other cell migration and invasion, cleaves endoglin from cell surfaces to release soluble endoglin.[162]
MMP 15	protease	MT-MMP; high concentration in syncytiotrophoblast of placenta, increases in pre-eclampsia.[163]

Tissue inhibitors of matrix metalloproteinases (TIMPs) are, as the name implies, proteins that directly inhibit the activity of the MMPs. There are four members of the TIMP family, TIMP 1, TIMP 2, TIMP 3, and TIMP 4.[164] TIMPs are produced by cells and secreted into the ECM, where they directly bind to the MMPs.[164] Cells use TIMPs for long range control since the MMPs are part of the ECM.

4.6 PROTEOGLYCANS

Proteoglycans are core proteins that are heavily glycosylated with glycosaminoglycan (GAG) sugar chains. GAGs are highly sulfated and negatively charged, resulting in a high osmotic potential and the ability to electrostatically bind growth factors.[165] Heparan sulfate proteoglycans have especially strong interactions with growth factors, retaining growth factors in the tissue matrix and protecting them from degradation.[166] Proteoglycans can aggregate by binding hyaluronan or collagen chains.[167] Common proteoglycans are described in the Table below.

Table III. Common proteoglycans and their associated GAGs and functions.

PROTEOGLYCAN	GLYCOSAMINOGLYCAN	FUNCTION
Decorin	Chondroitin sulfate & dermatan sulfate	Small leucine-rich proteoglycan (SLRP), component of connective tissue, binds collagen I fibrils, plays role in matrix assembly.[168, 169]
Biglycan	Chondroitin sulfate & dermatan sulfate	Small leucine-rich proteoglycan (SLRP), component of extracellular matrix in bone, cartilage, and tendon, interacts with collagen I and II, plays role in mineralization of bone.[170]
Versican	Chondroitin sulfate & dermatan sulfate	Large proteoglycan, present in many tissue including smooth muscle of blood vessels, epithelial cells of skin, and central and peripheral nervous system, has anti-adhesive properties and modulations inflammation.[171]
Perlecan	Heparan sulfate & chondroitin sulfate	Large proteoglycan, key component of vascular ECM, synthesized by vascular endothelial cells and smooth muscle cells, binds and crosslinks ECM components and cell surface markers.[172, 173]
Neurocan	Chondroitin sulfate	Primarily expressed in the central nervous system, modulates cell adhesion and migration, including neurite outgrowth.[174]
Aggrecan	Chondroitin sulfate	Major proteoglycan in cartilage, retains water and provides compressive strength.[167]
Fibromodulin	Keratan sulfate	Small interstitial proteoglycan, interacts with collagen I and II fibrils, plays role in assembly of ECM, inhibit fibrillogenesis.[168, 169, 175]

CHAPTER 5

MOLECULAR SIGNALS IN TISSUE REGENERATION AND HEALING

As described previously, cells communicate through a variety of physical and soluble signals. Cells can bind ECM and adhesion or cell surface regulatory molecules on neighboring cells, and they can respond to mechanical forces and physical contact. Cells also communicate through soluble autocrine and paracrine signaling by release or activation of cytokines, growth factors, hormones, steroids, enzymes, and other chemicals. As shown in Figure 22, autocrine signaling refers to when a cell secretes a factor which then binds receptors on that same cell, leading to a signaling response in that same cell. Paracrine signaling refers to when a cell secretes a factor which binds receptors on different cells nearby, leading to signaling responses in those neighboring cells. In contrast to local effectors, endocrine signaling refers to systemic secretion of factors into the bloodstream, with signaling to distant cells found downstream. Following release, signaling proteins can also electrostatically bind to ECM through charge interactions where they are stabilized until they are released by environmental changes, such as changes in pH or ECM degradation.

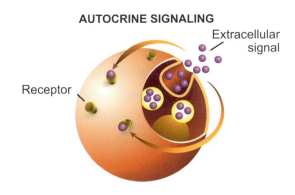

AUTOCRINE SIGNALING

Extracellular signal

Receptor

Target sites on same cell

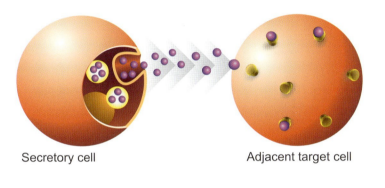

PARACRINE SIGNALING

Secretory cell

Adjacent target cell

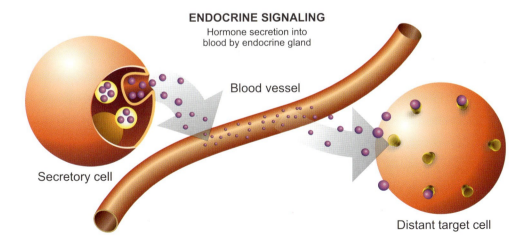

ENDOCRINE SIGNALING

Hormone secretion into blood by endocrine gland

Blood vessel

Secretory cell

Distant target cell

Figure 22. Autocrine signaling on the same cell, paracrine signaling to an adjacent cell, and endocrine signaling to a distant cell through the bloodstream.

When a molecule or ligand binds a receptor on a cell surface as shown in Figure 23, these signals stimulate a chain reaction or signaling cascade which alters cell behavior, often activating a series of molecules and signaling to the cell nucleus where it triggers responses at the gene expression level. These genes are transcribed into messenger RNA (mRNA) code which is then translated into the amino acid sequence that forms proteins, as in Figure 24. In this way, signaling molecules can both enhance and inhibit cellular activity, and through the multitude of complex signals cellular signals communicate to regulate cellular behavior.

Ligand-Receptor Signaling Cascade

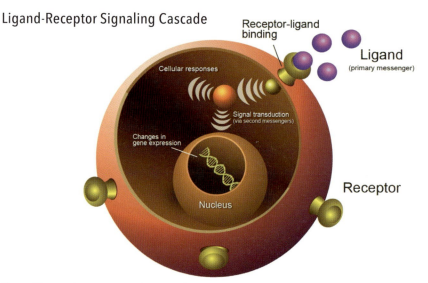

Figure 23. Ligand-receptor signaling cascade. Ligands bind receptors, which activate signaling cascades and then promote changes in gene expression in the nucleus.

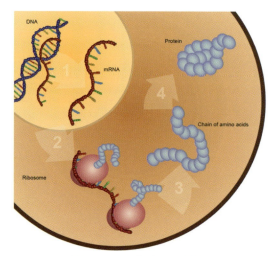

Figure 24. Gene expression process as 1) DNA is transcribed into mRNA, 2) mRNA is transported from the nucleus to the cytoplasm, 3) mRNA is translated by ribosomes to form a chain of amino acids, and 4) proteins fold into 3D conformations.

When discussing tissue healing, three classes of factors are essential to promote tissue regeneration: 1) immunomodulatory chemokines, 2) immunomodulatory cytokines, and 3) factors that promote tissue growth. *Immunomodulatory chemokines* influence the early inflammation stage of healing by recruiting reparative cells to the wounded tissue. *Immunomodulatory cytokines* regulate cellular response of the inflammatory cells at the wound to promote tissue repair. *Factors that promote tissue growth* then include growth factors, cytokines, hormones, and regulatory molecules that stimulate tissue growth through cell migration, proliferation, matrix production, additional cytokine signaling, and remodeling in the later stages of healing.

5.1 SIGNALING MOLECULES IN MIMEDX DEHYDRATED HUMAN AMNION/CHORION MEMBRANE (dHACM) ALLOGRAFTS

Previously, 57 growth factors and cytokines, including immunomodulatory chemokines, immunomodulatory cytokines, and tissue growth promoting factors, have been reported in dHACM tissue, as identified in Table IV below.[73-75]

Table IV. List of regulators of inflammation and soft tissue healing identified in dHACM.[73-75]

REGULATORS OF INFLAMMATION IN DHACM		REGULATORS OF SOFT TISSUE HEALING IN DHACM	
CYTOKINES	ABBREVIATION	CYTOKINES	ABBREVIATION
Granulocyte Colony-Stimulating Factor	GCSF	Angiogenin	Ang
Granulocyte Macrophage Colony-Stimulating Factor	GM-CSF	Angiopoietin-2	Ang-2
Growth Differentiation Factor 15	GDF-15	Basic Fibroblast Growth Factor	bFGF
Interferon Gamma	IFNγ	Bone Morphogenetic Protein 5	BMP-5
Interleukin 1 Alpha	IL-1α	Brain-Derived Neurotrophic Factor	BDNF
Interleukin 1 Beta	IL-1β	Endocrine Gland-Derived Vascular Endothelial Growth Factor	EG-VEGF
Interleukin 1 Receptor Antagonist	IL-1Ra	Epidermal Growth Factor	EGF
Interleukin 4	IL-4	Fibroblast Growth Factor 4	FGF-4
Interleukin 5	IL-5	Keratinocyte Growth Factor	KGF; FGF-7

REGULATORS OF INFLAMMATION IN dHACM		REGULATORS OF SOFT TISSUE HEALING IN dHACM	
CYTOKINES	**ABBREVIATION**	**CYTOKINES**	**ABBREVIATION**
Interleukin 6	IL-6	Growth Hormone	GH
Interleukin 7	IL-7	Heparin Binding EGF-Like Growth Factor	HB-EGF
Interleukin 10	IL-10	Hepatocyte Growth Factor	HGF
Interleukin 12 p40	IL-12p40	Insulin-Like Growth Factor 1	IGF-I
Interleukin 12 p70	IL-12p70	Insulin-Like Growth Factor Binding Protein 1	IGFBP-1
Interleukin 15	IL-15	Insulin-Like Growth Factor Binding Protein 2	IGFBP-2
Interleukin 17	IL-17	Insulin-Like Growth Factor Binding Protein 3	IGFBP-3
Macrophage Colony-Stimulating Factor	MCSF	Insulin-Like Growth Factor Binding Protein 4	IGFBP-4
Osteoprotegerin	OPG	Insulin-Like Growth Factor Binding Protein 6	IGFBP-6
CHEMOKINES	**ABBREVIATION**	Beta Nerve Growth Factor	β-NGF
B Lymphocyte Chemoattractant (CXCL13)	BLC	Placental Growth Factor	PlGF
Eotaxin 2	Eotaxin-2	Platelet-Derived Growth Factor AA	PDGF-AA
Chemokine Ligand 1 (CCL1)	I-309	Platelet-Derived Growth Factor BB	PDGF-BB
Interleukin 8	IL-8	Transforming Growth Factor Alpha	TGF-α
Interleukin 16	IL-16	Transforming Growth Factor Beta 1	TGF-β1
Monocyte Chemotactic Protein 1 (CCL2)	MCP-1	Vascular Endothelial Growth Factor	VEGF
Monokine Induced by Gamma Interferon (CXCL9)	MIG	**TISSUE INHIBITORS OF METALLOPROTEINASES**	**ABBREVIATION**
Macrophage Inflammatory Protein 1 Alpha (CCL3)	MIP-1α	Tissue Inhibitor of Metalloproteinases 1	TIMP-1
Macrophage Inflammatory Protein 1 Beta (CCL4)	MIP-1β	Tissue Inhibitor of Metalloproteinases 2	TIMP-2
Macrophage Inflammatory Protein 1D (MIP-5, CCL15)	MIP-1d	Tissue Inhibitor of Metalloproteinases 4	TIMP-4
Regulated on Activation, Normal T-cell Expressed and Secreted (CCL5)	RANTES		

5.1.1 IMMUNOMODULATORY CYTOKINES

Each of these regulatory factors possess distinct, yet overlapping cellular functions. A number of cytokines known to modulate inflammation were identified in dHACM. These immunomodulatory cytokines regulate leukocyte proliferation, differentiation, and activation to control the inflammatory response. Various functions of each are briefly described in Table V below.

Table V. Descriptions and functions of cytokine regulators of inflammation identified in dHACM.

CYTOKINE REGULATORS OF INFLAMMATION IN dHACM

CYTOKINES	FUNCTION
GCSF	Produced by macrophages, endothelial cells, fibroblasts, and other immune cells. Stimulates the proliferation, differentiation, survival, and activation of neutrophils. Promotes T cell polarization to a Th2 phenotype and production of regulatory dendritic cells.[176] Induces stem cell mobilization from bone marrow into peripheral blood.[177] Acts as a neurotrophic factor with roles in neuroprotection and neurogenesis.[178]
GM-CSF	Secreted by lymphocytes, macrophages, fibroblasts, endothelial cells, chondrocytes, and smooth muscle cells. Stimulates production and activation of neutrophils, and macrophages. Strengthens immune response and defends against infections.[179]
GDF-15	Mostly secreted in epithelial cells and macrophages, but also expressed in many tissues. Regulates inflammatory and apoptotic pathways in injured tissues. Inhibits macrophage activation,[180] and suppresses neutrophil adhesion and recruitment.[181] Has protective effects in cardiac tissue,[182] as well as neurotrophic effects.[183]
IFNγ	Produced predominantly by T cells and natural killer cells, as well as macrophages. Activates macrophages, promotes NK cell activity, and promotes Th1 differentiation. Increases expression of MHC class I and II. Stimulates response against viral and bacterial infections, and directly inhibits viral replication as well.[184]
IL-1α	Produced by macrophages, neutrophils, B cells, natural killer cells, as well as epithelial cells, endothelial cells, and fibroblasts. Promotes proliferation of keratinocytes, fibroblasts, smooth muscle cells, T cells, and B cells, as well as collagen synthesis. Maintains skin barrier function.[185-187]
IL-1β	Produced by a variety of cells and mediates inflammatory response, similar to IL-1α.[185-187]
IL-1Ra	Secreted by macrophages, neutrophils, epithelial cells, endothelial cells, and fibroblasts. Acts as an antagonist of IL-1 by binding IL-1 receptor and preventing IL-1 signaling.[188]
IL-4	Secreted by T cells, basophils, eosinophils, and mast cells. Induces differentiation of naïve helper T cells to Th2 cells and macrophages to M2 macrophages.[189, 190]
IL-5	Produced by T cells, eosinophils, and mast cells. Regulates proliferation, activation, differentiation, survival, and adhesion of eosinophils. Involved in tissue remodeling and wound healing.[190]
IL-6	Secreted by macrophages, fibroblasts, and endothelial cells. Has both pro-inflammatory and anti-inflammatory effects. Stimulates growth, differentiation, and activation of T and B cells to fight infection and stimulate the immune response after trauma.[190] Also inhibits TNF-a and IL-1,[191] and activates expression of IL-1Ra and IL-10.[192]

CYTOKINE REGULATORS OF INFLAMMATION IN dHACM

CYTOKINES	FUNCTION
IL-7	Secreted by epithelial cells, keratinocytes, dendritic cells, macrophages, and B cells. Stimulates proliferation, maturation, and survival of B cells, T cells, and natural killer cells.[190]
IL-10	Produced in monocytes and lymphocytes, T cells, B cells, mast cells, natural killer cells, and dendritic cells. Regulates growth and differentiation of B cells, natural killer cells, T cells, mast cells, granulocytes, dendritic cells, keratinocytes, and endothelial cells. Promotes differentiation of Th2 cells and M2 macrophages, and inhibits expression of cytokines by T cells and macrophages, including IL-1, IFN-γ, and TNF-α.[193]
IL-12p40	Beta subunit of IL-12. Acts as IL-12p70 antagonist by binding IL-12 receptor. Also acts as a chemoattractant for macrophages and dendritic cells.[194]
IL-12p70	Active heterodimer of IL-12. Produced by macrophages, neutrophils, dendritic cells, and B cells. Stimulates growth and differentiation to Th1 cells.[190]
IL-15	Produced by monocytes, macrophages, T cells, keratinocytes, and fibroblasts. Stimulates proliferation and activation of T lymphocytes and natural killer cells.[190]
IL-17	Produced by T cells, neutrophils, natural killer cells, as well as epithelial cells, endothelial cells, fibroblasts. Increases production of cytokines, chemokines, and MMPs to recruit monocytes and neutrophils to sites of inflammation.[190]
MCSF	Produced by macrophages, natural killer cells, B and T cells, fibroblasts, epithelial cells, endothelial cells, keratinocytes, and osteoblasts. Simulates HSC differentiation to monocytes and macrophages. Involved in proliferation, differentiation, activation, and survival of monocytes and macrophages.[195]
OPG	Soluble decoy receptor that inhibits receptor activation of NFkB ligation (RANKL) to regulate inflammation, cell survival, and differentiation. Inhibits production, differentiation, and activation of osteoclasts, as well as proliferation, activation, and cytokine secretion by T cells and dendritic cells.[196, 197]

5.1.2 IMMUNOMODULATORY CHEMOKINES

A number of chemokines known to modulate inflammation were identified in dHACM. These immunomodulatory chemokines act as chemoattractants to recruit leukocyte migration toward injured tissues. Various functions of each are briefly described in Table VI below.

Table VI. Descriptions and functions of chemokine regulators of inflammation identified in dHACM.

CHEMOKINE REGULATORS OF INFLAMMATION IN dHACM

CHEMOKINES	FUNCTION
BLC	Mostly secreted in T cells. Selectively chemotactic for B lymphocytes.[198]
Eotaxin-2	Induces chemotaxis in eosinophils, T lymphocytes, and neutrophils.[199, 200]
I-309	Secreted by T cells. Recruits monocytes, natural killer cells, B cells, and dendritic cells.[201, 202]
IL-8	Produced by macrophages, epithelial cells, smooth muscle cells, and endothelial cells. Induces chemotaxis in neutrophils and other granulocytes. Induces phagocytosis and promotes angiogenesis.[203, 204]
IL-16	Released by a variety of cells including lymphocytes and epithelial cells. Chemoattractant for CD4+ cells, including T cells, monocytes, eosinophils, and dendritic cells.[205, 206]
MCP-1	Secreted by monocytes, macrophages, and dendritic cells, as well as osteoblasts, neurons, astrocytes, and microglia. Recruits monocytes, memory T cells, and dendritic cells.[207, 208]
MIG	Chemoattractant for T cells.[209]
MIP-1α	Secreted by macrophages, dendritic cells, and lymphocytes. Chemotactic for neutrophils and monocytes.[210]
MIP-1β	Secreted by macrophages, dendritic cells, and lymphocytes. Chemoattractant for natural killer cells, monocytes, and other immune cells.[210]
MIP-1δ	Secreted by macrophages, dendritic cells, and lymphocytes. Chemoattractant for neutrophils, monocytes, and lymphocytes.[210]
RANTES	Secreted by T cells and other immune cells. Chemotactic for T cells, eosinophils, and monocytes.[211]

5.1.3 TISSUE GROWTH PROMOTING FACTORS

A number of cytokines known to promote tissue growth were identified in dHACM. These tissue growth promoting factors regulate cell migration, proliferation, ECM production and remodeling, as well as angiogenesis. Various functions of each are briefly described in Table VII below.

Table VII. Descriptions and functions of cytokine regulators of soft tissue healing identified in dHACM.

TISSUE GROWTH PROMOTING REGULATORS OF SOFT TISSUE HEALING IN dHACM

CYTOKINES	FUNCTION
Ang	Potent stimulator of angiogenesis. Stimulates migration, proliferation, and vessel formation by endothelial and smooth muscle cells. Has ribonuclease activity, which alters gene expression and protein synthesis. Activates proteases that degrade laminin and fibronectin in basement membrane, allowing vessel formation.[212]
Ang-2	Regulates neovascularization in conjunction with angiopoeitin-1 and VEGF. When signaling in conjunction with VEGF, promotes neovascularization by promoting proliferation and migration of endothelial cells.[213] Without VEGF, acts as an antagonist to angiopoietin-1 signaling by promoting endothelial cell death and disrupting vascularization.[214]
bFGF	Heparin-binding protein with broad mitogenic activity in a wide variety of cells; Potent stimulator of angiogenesis; Regulates differentiation of stem cells and tissue development.[215]
BMP-5	Expressed in the nervous system, lungs, and liver; Regulates bone and cartilage development, growth, and remodeling; Regulates dendrite growth in neurons.[216]
BDNF	Expressed in many tissues including the brain; Supports the growth, differentiation, and survival of neurons through neurogenesis.[217]
EG-VEGF	Secreted by liver and kidney endothelial cells, and involved in placental development; stimulates endothelial cell migration, proliferation, and survival; Potent stimulator of angiogenesis.[218, 219]
EGF	Stimulates proliferation, differentiation, and survival in numerous cell types, including epithelial cells.[220]
FGF-4	Broad mitogenic and cell survival activity; involved in development, cell growth, morphogenesis, and tissue repair.[221, 222]
KGF; FGF-7	Heparin-binding protein; Produced during epithelialization phase of wound healing; Promotes proliferation and migration of epithelial cells and keratinocytes.[223]
GH	Peptide hormone secreted by pituitary gland; Stimulates body growth through IGF-1 production; Involved in anabolic activity, including increased protein synthesis, tissue growth, and immune response.[224]
HB-EGF	Heparin binding growth factor produced by monocytes and macrophages; Regulates cell adhesion, proliferation, migration, and survival; Causes keratinocytes and fibroblasts to migrate to the wound and proliferate; Promotes angiogenesis.[225, 226]

TISSUE GROWTH PROMOTING REGULATORS OF SOFT TISSUE HEALING IN dHACM

CYTOKINES	FUNCTION
HGF	Secreted by mesenchymal cells; Regulates cell growth, cell motility, and morphogenesis in epithelial cells and endothelial cells; Stimulates angiogenesis.[227]
IGF-I	Hormone produced by liver; Stimulates body growth through broad mitogenic activity in nearly every cell type.[224]
IGFBP-1	Expressed in nearly all tissues; Binds and stabilizes IGF-1 as a carrier protein; Regulates IGF-1 activity.[228]
IGFBP-2	Expressed in nearly all tissues; Binds and stabilizes IGF-1 as a carrier protein; Regulates IGF-1 activity.[228]
IGFBP-3	Expressed in nearly all tissues; Binds and stabilizes IGF-1 as a carrier protein; Regulates IGF-1 activity.[228]
IGFBP-4	Expressed in nearly all tissues; Binds and stabilizes IGF-1 as a carrier protein; Regulates IGF-1 activity.[228]
IGFBP-6	Expressed in nearly all tissues; Binds and stabilizes IGF-1 as a carrier protein; Regulates IGF-1 activity.[228]
β-NGF	Important for promoting growth, maintenance, and survival of neurons.[229]
PlGF	Simulates proliferation and migration of endothelial cells; Potent stimulator of angiogenesis.[230]
PDGF-AA	Stimulates proliferation and migration of mesenchymal cells; Promotes angiogenesis during tissue development and within healing wounds.[231, 232]
PDGF-BB	Stimulates proliferation and migration of mesenchymal cells; Promotes angiogenesis during tissue development and within healing wounds.[231, 232]
TGF-α	Produced by macrophages, brain cells, and keratinocytes; Stimulates proliferation and migration of keratinocytes; Promotes angiogenesis during tissue development and within healing wounds.[233, 234]
TGF-β1	Secreted by many cell types, including macrophages; Controls proliferation, differentiation, and apoptosis of numerous cell types.[235]
VEGF	Stimulates endothelial cell migration and activation; Potent stimulator of angiogenesis; Chemotactic for macrophages and granulocytes.[236]
TIMP-1	Binds and inactivates a number of matrix metalloproteinases (MMPs) to inhibit tissue degradation.[164]
TIMP-2	Binds and inactivates a number of matrix metalloproteinases (MMPs) to inhibit tissue degradation.[164]
TIMP-4	Binds and inactivates a number of matrix metalloproteinases (MMPs) to inhibit tissue degradation.[164]

5.1.4 A TOTAL OF 226 KNOWN REGULATORS OF HEALING AND INFLAMMATION HAVE BEEN IDENTIFIED IN MIMEDX dHACM

In addition to the 57 previously reported regulators of healing and inflammation described above, an additional 169 regulator molecules have recently been identified in MiMedx PURION Processed dHACM allografts.[237] Similarly, these 169 additional factors, which are listed in Table VIII below, include immunomodulatory chemokines, immunomodulatory cytokines, and tissue growth promoting factors that play various roles in regulating soft tissue healing and inflammation. With the addition of these factors, **226 growth factors, cytokines, and regulator molecules that modulate healing and inflammation have been identified in MiMedx PURION Processed dHACM allografts** to date.

Table VIII. Additional 169 regulators of healing and inflammation which have been recently identified in dHACM.[237]

CYTOKINES	ABBREVIATION	CYTOKINES	ABBREVIATION
6Ckine (CCL21)	6Ckine	Angiotensinogen	Angiotensinogen
A Disintegrin and Metalloproteinase with Thrombospondin Type 1 Motif 13	ADAMTS13	B-Cell Activating Factor	BAFF
A Proliferation-Inducing Ligand	APRIL	Betacellulin	BTC
Acidic Fibroblast Growth Factor	aFGF	Bone Morphogenetic Protein 2	BMP-2
Activin A	Activin A	Bone Morphogenetic Protein 7	BMP-7
Adiponectin	Adiponectin	Bone Morphogenetic Protein 9	BMP-9
Adipsin	Adipsin	C-Reactive Protein	CRP
Agouti-Related Protein	AgRP	C-X-C Motif Chemokine Ligand 14	CXCL14
Angiopoietin-1	ANG-1	C-X-C Motif Chemokine Ligand 16	CXCL16
Angiopoietin-4	ANG-4	Carbonic Anhydrase 9	CA9
Angiopoietin-Like 3	ANGPTL3	Carcinoembryonic Antigen	CEA
Angiopoietin-Like 4	ANGPTL4	Chemerin	Chemerin
Angiostatin	Angiostatin	Chemerin	Chemerin
Angiotensin Converting Enzyme 2	ACE-2	Chitinase-3-Like Protein 1	CHI3L1

CYTOKINES	ABBREVIATION	CYTOKINES	ABBREVIATION
Ciliary Neurotrophic Factor	CNTF	Follicle-Stimulating Hormone	FSH
Ck Beta 8-1 (CCL23)	Ck beta 8-1	Follistatin	Follistatin
Clusterin	Clusterin	Follistatin-Like 1	Follistatin-like 1
Coagulation Factor XIV	CF XIV	Follistatin-Related Gene	FLRG
Complement Component 5a	C5a	Fractalkine	Fractalkine
Cripto-1	Cripto-1	Furin	Furin
Cystatin A	Cystatin A	G-Protein Coupled Receptor-Associated Sorting Protein 1	GASP-1
Cystatin B	Cystatin B	G-Protein Coupled Receptor-Associated Sorting Protein 2 (WFIKKN)	GASP-2
Cystatin C	Cystatin C	Galectin-1	Galectin-1
Cystatin Endogenous Marker	Cystatin E M	Galectin-2	Galectin-2
Deadenylating Nuclease	DAN	Galectin-3	Galectin-3
Decoy Receptor 3	DcR3	Galectin-7	Galectin-7
Delta-Like Protein 1	DLL1	Galectin-9	Galectin-9
Dickkopf-Related Protein 1	DKK-1	Glial Cell Line-Derived Neurotrophic Factor	GDNF
Dickkopf-Related Protein 3	Dkk-3	Glycoprotein 130	gp130
Dickkopf-Related Protein 4	Dkk-4	Granulocyte Chemotactic Protein 2 (CXCL6)	GCP-2
Eotaxin	Eotaxin	Granulysin	Granulysin
Eotaxin-3	Eotaxin-3	Growth Arrest-Specific Protein 1	Gas 1
Epithelial-Derived Neutrophil-Activating Protein 78 (CXCL5)	ENA-78	Growth-Regulated Alpha Protein (CXCL1)	GROα
Fatty Acid-Binding Protein 2	FABP2	Growth-Regulated Protein	GRO
Fetuin A	Fetuin A	Hemofiltrate C-C Motif Chemokine 1 (CCL14)	HCC-1
Fibroblast Growth Factor 6	FGF-6	Hepatocyte Growth Factor Activator Inhibitor Type 2	HAI-2
Fibroblast Growth Factor 9	FGF-9	Human Chorionic Gonadotropin Beta	hCGβ
Fibroblast Growth Factor 19	FGF-19	Insulin	Insulin
Fibroblast Growth Factor 21	FGF-21	Insulin-Like Growth Factor 2	IGF-2
Fms-Related Tyrosine Kinase 3 Ligand	Flt-3L	Insulin-Like Growth Factor Binding Protein 5	IGFBP-5

CYTOKINES	ABBREVIATION	CYTOKINES	ABBREVIATION
Interferon Gamma-Induced Protein 10 (CXCL10)	IP-10	Interleukin 33	IL-33
Interferon-Inducible T-Cell Alpha Chemoattractant (CXCL11)	I-TAC	Interleukin 34	IL-34
Interleukin 1 Family Member 5 (IL-36ra)	IL-1 F5	Kallikrein 5	Kallikrein 5
Interleukin 1 Family Member 6 (IL-36α)	IL-1 F6	Kallikrein 14	Kallikrein 14
Interleukin 1 Family Member 7 (IL-37)	IL-1 F7	Latency-Associated Peptide Transforming Growth Factor Beta 1	LAP(TGFb1)
Interleukin 1 Family Member 8 (IL-36β)	IL-1 F8	Legumain	Legumain
Interleukin 1 Family Member 9 (IL-36γ)	IL-1 F9	Leptin	Leptin
Interleukin 1 Family Member 10 (IL-38)	IL-1 F10	Leucine-Rich Repeats and Immunoglobulin-Like Domains 3	LRIG3
Interleukin 1 Receptor-Like 1	ST2	Lipocalin-2	Lipocalin-2
Interleukin 2	IL-2	Lymphotactin	Lymphotactin
Interleukin 3	IL-3	Macrophage Migration Inhibitory Factor	MIF
Interleukin 6 Soluble Receptor	IL-6sR	Mannose-Binding Lectin	MBL
Interleukin 8	IL-8	Marapsin	Marapsin
Interleukin 11	IL-11	Midkine	Midkine
Interleukin 17B	IL-17B	Monocyte Chemotactic Protein 2 (CCL8)	MCP-2
Interleukin 17C	IL-17C	Nephroblastoma Overexpressed (CCN3)	NOV
Interleukin 17E (IL25)	IL-17E	Neuregulin 1	NRG1-β1
Interleukin 20	IL-20	Neuron-Specific Enolase	NSE
Interleukin 21	IL-21	Neurotrophin-3	NT-3
Interleukin 23	IL-23	Neurotrophin-4	NT-4
Interleukin 24	IL-24	Neutrophil-Activating Protein 2 (CXCL7)	NAP-2
Interleukin 27	IL-27	Oncostatin M	OSM
Interleukin 32 Alpha	IL-32α	Osteoactivin	Osteoactivin

CYTOKINES	ABBREVIATION	CYTOKINES	ABBREVIATION
Osteopontin	OPN	Thrombospondin 1	TSP-1
Pentraxin-Related Protein 3	PTX 3	Thrombospondin-2	Thrombospondin-2
Peptidoglycan Recognition Protein Short	PGRP-S	Thrombospondin-5	Thrombospondin-5
Plasminogen Activator Inhibitor-1	PAI-1	Thyroglobulin	Thyroglobulin
Platelet-Derived Growth Factor AB	PDGF-AB	Thyroid Stimulating Hormone	TSH
Platelet Factor 4 (CXCL4)	PF4	Tissue Factor Pathway Inhibitor	TFPI
Preadipocyte Factor 1	Pref-1	Transforming Growth Factor Beta 2	TGFb2
Procalcitonin	Procalcitonin	Transforming Growth Factor Beta 3	TGFb3
Prolactin	Prolactin	Transforming Growth Factor Beta-Induced Protein ig-H3	βIG-H3
Pulmonary and Activation-Regulated Chemokine (CCL18)	PARC	Trappin-2	Trappin-2
Pulmonary Surfactant-Associated Protein D	SP-D	Tumor Necrosis Factor Alpha	TNF-α
Renin	Renin	Tumor Necrosis Factor Beta	TNF-β
Repulsive Guidance Molecule Domain Family Member B	RGM-B	Tumor Necrosis Factor Ligand Superfamily Member 14	LIGHT
Resistin	Resistin	Tumor Necrosis Factor-Related Activation-Induced Cytokine	TRANCE
Retinol-Binding Protein 4	RBP4	Tumor Necrosis Factor-Related Apoptosis-Inducing Ligand	TRAIL
S100 Calcium-Binding Protein A8	S100A8	Tumor Necrosis Factor-Related Weak Inducer of Apoptosis	TWEAK
Secreted Frizzled-Related Protein 3	sFRP-3	UL16-Binding Protein 1	ULBP-1
Serpin A4	Serpin A4	Uterine-Specific Proline-Rich Acidic Protein	uPA
Sonic Hedgehog N-Terminal	Shh-N	Vascular Endothelial Growth Factor C	VEGF-C
Stem Cell Factor	SCF	Vascular Endothelial Growth Factor D	VEGF-D
Stromal Cell-Derived Factor 1 Beta	SDF-1β	Wnt Inhibitory Factor 1	WIF-1
Thrombopoietin	TPO	Wnt1-Inducible-Signaling Pathway Protein 1 (CCN4)	WISP-1

The relative content of factors identified in MiMedx PURION Processed dHACM is shown graphically in Figure 25. Due to the complexity of this unique material, significant research would be required over a lengthy period of time to fully elucidate the functional roles of each of these molecules in mediating healing; therefore, at this time, a causative effect cannot be assigned to any single regulatory protein either currently identified or yet to be identified in dHACM tissues. However, all of the molecules present in dHACM allografts likely act synergistically and in a critical balance of regulatory signals to promote healing, as observed clinically with MiMedx dHACM tissues.[47, 80-94]

Angiostatin	IGFBP-3	ACE-2	Adiponectin	Pref-1	Fetuin A
Galectin-7	Thyroglobulin	NSE	TSP-1	Follistatin-like 1	ANGPTL4
TIMP-2	OPN	PAI-1	Angiotensinogen	gp130	IGFBP-5
IL-1 F10	Furin	IL-1 F5	Serpin A4	RBP4	Adipsin
IGFBP-2	DKK-1	IL-1 F7	Midkine	hCGb	TIMP-1
FLRG	GROa	Gas 1	TGFb1	Legumain	LRIG3
IGFBP-6	PF4	CRP	IL-1 F6	Prolactin	IGFBP-1
Pentraxin 3	BMP-5	HGF	Dkk-3	bIG-H3	BMP-2
Resistin	Granulysin	6Ckine	IL-1 F9	RANTES	HAI-2
CA9	Galectin-1	EG-VEGF	Osteoactivin	WIF-1	CXCL14
OSM	DAN	Cystatin B	DcR3	Galectin-3	IGFBP-4
TRAIL	IL-21	CHI3L1	Fractalkine	Follistatin	FSH
Thrombospondin-5	Clusterin	IL-17C	LAP(TGFb1)	APRIL	TRANCE
WISP-1	MIF	SP-D	IGF-2	Insulin	TWEAK
S100A8	GDF-15	uPA	DLL1	IL-24	Galectin-9
RGM-B	CEA	ANG-4	PDGF-BB	CF XIV	ADAMTS13
Marapsin	MIP-1a	Shh-N	Angiogenin	ULBP-1	ANG-2
PGRP-S	CXCL16	TSH	Cystatin A	Chemerin	MCP-2
Thrombospondin-2	CNTF	Renin	BMP-7	C5a	IL-27
aFGF	TPO	NT-4	MBL	MIG	HCC-1
FABP2	Procalcitonin	GASP-2	Cystatin E M	IL-23	Kallikrein 14
OPG	sFRP-3	ANGPTL3	NOV	IL-17B	bFGF
Trappin-2	FGF-19	FGF-6	Eotaxin-3	VEGF-C	ANG-1
Dkk-4	PDGF-AA	NAP-2	PDGF-AB	IL-6sR	IL-16
Lipocalin-2	MCP-1	BDNF	IL-33	MIP-1b	IL-11
Cystatin C	Kallikrein 5	ST2	SDF-1b	ENA-78	BLC
FGF-9	PARC	IL-34	IL-6	IL-20	IL-17E
IL-1ra	FGF-21	BAFF	BMP-9	TGFb2	TIMP-4
Leptin	VEGF	EGF	LIGHT	Lymphotactin	IL-3
MCSF	IP-10	GH	TNFb	AgRP	Galectin-2
Cripto-1	NT-3	IGF-I	IL-1a	TNFa	SCF
GASP-1	IL-18	BTC	NRG1-b1	I-TAC	GCP-2
TFPI	IL-8	TGFb3	FGF-7	Flt-3L	GM-CSF
GRO	IL-1 F8	MIP-1d	IL-32 alpha	IL-1b	Activin A
GDNF	VEGF-D	Ck beta 8-1	IL-7	G-CSF	IL-15
PIGF	I-309	IL-12p40	HB-EGF	IL-2	IL-4
Eotaxin-2	Eotaxin				

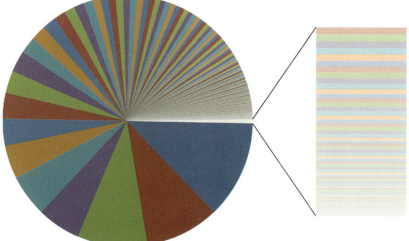

Figure 25. Graphical depiction of the relative contents of various growth factors, cytokines, and regulatory molecules identified in dHACM.

5.2 DYNAMIC RECIPROCITY IN CELL SIGNALING

Human tissues consist of three fundamental components: extracellular matrix (ECM); protein growth factors, cytokines, and chemokine molecules bound to the ECM; and living cells. Each is required for tissue healing to occur following an injury. Changes in the levels or condition of any one of these components of a tissue following injury lead to reciprocal responses from the other two components to restore the tissue to a state of normality and balance (homeostasis), which we recognize as the outcome of tissue repair or healing. Application of external mechanical forces, such as tension across skin or load applied to bone, also act as important physical signals to cells to stimulate tissue repair, and contribute as a fourth component in addition to the ECM, growth factors/ cytokine signaling molecules and cells required for healing.[238] These interactions in tissues are known as "dynamic reciprocity,"[238] and have been proposed to be operative across a variety of different tissue types. The general model is shown in Figure 26.

Dynamic Reciprocity

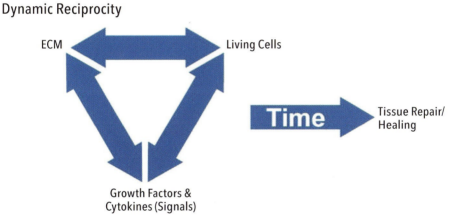

Figure 26. Illustration of the ECM, protein factors and living cellular components of tissues, and the interactions of the components involved in "dynamic reciprocity" that leads to normal tissue repair and healing.

A simpler way to think about this is to consider the ECM of a tissue as the framework of a house, and when the framework is damaged in a storm (injury), fragments of the framework (ECM) and the house alarm system (growth factors/ cytokine molecules), act as signals to recruit a team of workers (cells) to the affected area to fix the house and restore it back to its original, intact state. The recruited workers (cells) in turn release more alarm signals (growth factors/ cytokines) to help coordinate the repair of the tissue by replacing the framework (new ECM), modulating the debris cleanup crew (inflammatory response), regenerate the plumbing (angiogenesis), and restore the house as closely as possible back to its normal state (healed tissues).

Disease states, such as diabetes, lead to disruptions in the normal interactions between ECM, cells and growth factor/ cytokine molecules that may in part result in wounds that do not heal.[238] In other instances, patients may suffer from disease conditions that require treatment with aggressive medications that also affect the normal healing of tissues. In these instances, healing of injured tissues may benefit from treatment with dHACM that works to help restore some of the normal dynamic reciprocity in the affected tissue by way of providing a preserved ECM, and a complex array of soluble growth factors/ cytokines that recruit host cells to the site of the injury thereby stimulating progression towards healing.

Single growth factors are not representative of clinical outcomes, because growth factors, cytokines and chemokines possess redundancy of function to allow for compensation due to donor-to-donor and tissue-to-tissue variability.

This redundancy of function in growth factor signaling was developed over many years through the evolutionary process. Human evolution can be traced through the fossil record to the emergence of the first hominid primates six million years ago.[239] Along with other mammals, primates, including humans, evolved to give birth to live offspring, known as viviparous birth wherein fetal development occurs inside of the mother in an amniotic cavity enclosed by an amniotic sac. Thus, viviparous birth is a highly successful adaptation which over millions of years of evolution has resulted in the biochemically complex amniotic membrane occurring in humans today that acts as a protective barrier between the developing fetus and the mother, and which undergoes the proprietary PURION Processing to yield MiMedx's dHACM products, EpiFix and AmnioFix. In dHACM to date, we have been able to detect over 226 soluble protein growth factor, cytokine, and chemokine molecules that are natural constituents of amniotic tissue.[73-75,237] However, it is more likely that the number of different molecular factors residing in the tissue number in the hundreds or thousands,[240-242] each bound to the ECM making up a complex array of biologically active molecules that are advantageous to have immediately available to accelerate healing in case of injury to the membrane under natural conditions. We are only limited in being able to measure each and every one of these in dHACM by the availability of analytical tools and methodologies for the detection of each of these molecules.

Cytokines and chemokines are multifunctional in terms of their impact on cells, but many of these molecules residing in tissues play overlapping, redundant roles in biological systems. It is thought that this redundancy of function among cytokines has evolved to impart robustness and fine-tuning of cellular responses to tissue injury.[241,242] For example, the immunomodulatory molecules interleukin-2 (IL-2), IL-3, IL-5, and IL-9 have all been shown to stimulate proliferation of T-cells, which are white blood cells involved in the immune response,[240] demonstrating their functional redundancy in this role. Thus in

66

theory, if one of these molecules happened to be present in lower quantities than the others in any given sample of amniotic tissue, the action of the other interleukin molecules to stimulate T-cell proliferation may compensate for the deficiency of the one. Given this inherent redundancy among cytokines in tissues, such as amniotic tissue, it is unlikely that the neutralization of one cytokine would significantly interfere with the overall clinical outcome of tissue repair observed, for instance, during wound healing. It is likely that the totality of biological stimulation by the many factors present in complex tissues, and the built-in redundancy of their functions, that better ensures the positive tissue repair outcomes observed in treated patients in the clinic as opposed to the action of one or another of these factors.

In the case of angiogenesis, a critical process required for tissue repair, VEGF is an important factor for recruiting and stimulating endothelial cells to the site of injury, however, other factors also play critical roles in this process including FGF-2, PDGF-BB, TGF-β, and angiopoietin.[33] Overlapping roles for stimulating angiogenesis exist for VEGF and HGF.[243] Both FGF-2 and PDGF-BB stimulate recruitment of pericyte cells (smooth muscle cells) to new capillaries to stabilize them during angiogenesis.[244] These factors may compensate for one another in tissues to stimulate angiogenesis, and fluctuations in levels of one factor from tissue to tissue seem highly unlikely to impact the overall biological outcome of new blood vessel formation during healing. The likelihood that variability in tissue concentrations of any one of these factors correlating with observed clinical outcomes of tissue repair is likely remote given the biological complexity and robustness of human tissues, such as amniotic tissue as an example. The complexity, redundancy and compensatory properties of growth factors and cytokines found in human tissues has evolved to provide back-up systems to ensure healing, ultimately increasing the chances of survival for the individual.[238,242] Based on our current understanding of dHACM with the diversity and complexity of growth factors it contains, it is more likely that the totality of the factors added to an injured tissue and the diversity of biological responses they stimulate to re-establish the normal interactions of cells and ECM, results in the positive clinical outcomes we observe in the clinic following dHACM treatment of injured tissues.

CHAPTER 6

IN VITRO TECHNIQUES TO EXAMINE CELLULAR ACTIVITY

In order to analyze the effectiveness of dHACM grafts and to gather an abundance of information regarding the molecular mechanisms of action that are important to promote tissue healing and regeneration, MiMedx utilizes a variety of *in vitro* techniques to investigate biological activity of its PURION Processed dHACM products. *In vitro* experiments are used as simplified models to test the effects of experimental conditions within highly controlled environments. These *in vitro* models are used to test experimental hypotheses and provide significant knowledge of how dHACM products may influence cellular responses when implanted within clinically relevant wounds. *In vitro* techniques used by MiMedx involve characterization of the structure and content of dHACM grafts, as well as the cellular responses of various cells when treated with dHACM grafts.

6.1 PREVENTION OF "PSEUDOSCIENCE"

Due to the complexity of biological systems and the physiological healing response, scientifically sound experimental design is of critical importance to achieve meaningful scientific conclusions. The *scientific method* involves hypothesis-based experimentation, where only a single experimental condition is tested at a given time to support or reject a hypothesis. If more than one condition is changed at a given time, then the resulting effect cannot be attributed to any single condition, and conclusions cannot be made.

An essential component of the scientific method includes use of proper experimental controls, which provide appropriate comparisons to minimize the effects of unanticipated variables and increases the reliability of results. Experimental controls will tell the user if the experiments worked reliably and whether treatment conditions stimulated a specific cellular response. The *in vitro* experimental techniques utilized by MiMedx, including proper use of positive and negative controls, are discussed in the following sections of Chapter 6. Further discussion of *in vivo* animal models will be discussed in detail in Chapter 7, while proper design of clinical trials is discussed in Chapter 8.

Without scientifically sound experimental design, analytical techniques, interpretation, and validation of results, scientific conclusions may be misinterpreted. This approach to poorly conducted research may lead to false and deceptive results and should be viewed as *pseudoscience*. Pseudoscientific publications are the result. This is a disservice to clinicians and scientists who are truly attempting to substantiate the attributes of promising new tissue and cell technologies in regenerative medicine.

For example, normal cellular activity and healing are known to require a complex **balance of signals** to proceed naturally, including a balance of MMPs that degrade ECM and TIMPs that conversely inhibit MMP activity. All cells produce MMPs and TIMPs during normal tissue maintenance and healing, including proliferation, migration, differentiation, cell signaling, angiogenesis, and tissue remodeling.[34,35] Additionally, the MiMedx PURION Process has been shown to retain the native bioactivity of amniotic membrane by preserving **significantly more of the growth factors, cytokines, and regulatory proteins that are naturally present in amniotic tissues**, including both MMPs and their TIMP inhibitors, than amniotic membrane allografts that are processed using alternative techniques.[76,105,106] Therefore, it would be deceptive to suggest that PURION Processed tissues contain a higher content of "destructive" MMPs without also discussing the presence of TIMPs, which are present in excess in PURION Processed amniotic membrane allografts,[107,108] to demonstrate the balance of MMP activity and inhibition by TIMPs, as well as the natural role of MMPs and TIMPs in normal tissue maintenance and repair.

6.2 DESIGN OF *IN VITRO* CELL EXPERIMENTS

A cell is the smallest unit of life which is the structural and biological building block of all other living organisms. To examine the biological activity of various materials, experimental techniques have been developed to analyze cellular responses *in vitro* (Latin for "in glass"), or in the laboratory. Using aseptic technique in a laminar flow cabinet, in which air flow is microfiltered and carefully controlled to maintain sterility of the cabinet's contents, adherent cells can be cultured on glass or plastic materials, and nonadherent cells can be cultured in suspension in liquid solutions.

Because cells are alive, they have a metabolism and require nutrients. During *in vitro* cell culture studies, these nutrients are provided by a liquid or gel called culture medium. Culture medium is a neutral pH and isotonic environment of salts, amino acids and sugars to which soluble components are added to sustain or stimulate growth, or induce differentiation of cells. Each cell type has its own specific formulation of media for sustenance or differentiation. Also added to media is an essential amino acid called L-Glutamine. L-Glutamine is used to support the division of high activity cells by providing an alternate energy source *in vitro*. Some cell types require additional additives, such as sera, or various factors (e.g., defined growth factors, attachment factors, vitamins) for survival and growth. Culture media also often contain an antibiotic agent, commonly penicillin/streptomycin (pen/strep) or gentamicin, which is added to prevent the microbiological contamination of cells. Media plus its additives are known as complete media. Prior to use in seeding, feeding, or culturing cells, the media are warmed to 37°C, which is body temperature, for subsequent growth incubation. Every 2 to 3 days, culture medium is replenished with fresh media to remove cellular waste and replace depleted nutrients. Approximately once per week, depending on the cell type, seeding density, and population doubling times, the cells are subcultured (or "split") as a next passage to expand the population to larger numbers.

Cellular characteristics can be measured using a variety of analytical techniques. *In vitro* experiments allow cells and biological molecules to be studied outside of their natural environment. All experiments require both a negative and a positive control. *A negative control* is a treatment in which no response or only a baseline response is expected, as opposed to a *positive control* in which a known response is expected. As exemplified in Figure 27, the positive control compared to the negative control is used as evidence that the experiment did indeed work (Figure 27, left panel). If there is no response from the positive control, as in the right panel in Figure 27, then the experimental design must be reevaluated. A negative control is used as evidence that the experiment worked correctly in combination with the positive control and can also be used to qualify the response from the treatment groups in question, as in Figure 28. Any difference between the treatment groups and the negative control can be regarded as a result of the treatment, provided that the positive control works and affirms the study.

For instance:

Positive Control

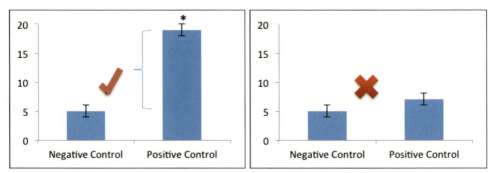

Figure 27. Examples of comparative outcomes in assay controls. A statistically significant positive response is expected in the Positive Control to determine whether the experiment performed as expected as demonstrated in the left panel (* indicates p≤0.05, compared to negative control). However, if the positive control does not demonstrate a statistically significant positive response, as in the right panel, this suggests that the assay may not have worked correctly, and further conclusions cannot be drawn from the experiment.

Negative Control

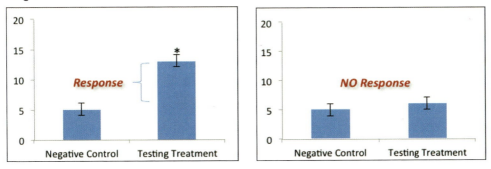

Figure 28. Examples of negative controls compared to test groups. Little or no response is expected in the Negative Control to determine whether the experiment performed as expected. If a testing condition demonstrates a statistically significant response, as demonstrated in the left panel (* indicates $p \leq 0.05$, compared to negative control), then the response can be attributed to the effects of the testing treatment. However, if the testing condition does not demonstrate a statistically significant response, as in the right panel, then no response can be attributed to the effects of the testing treatment.

In the case of cell based experiments, the negative control is most commonly basal media. *Basal media* is culture media which contains salts, amino acids, sugars, and other factors that will sustain cells for some time, but will not promote growth. Most commonly its formulation additives only include the addition of antibiotic(s) and L-glutamine. In order for the cells to replicate effectively, a serum supplement or specific growth factors must be added to the media. Serum is isolated from the coagulated blood of an animal, commonly fetal or other bovine serum, and has a rich variety of proteins which promote cell growth. This supplemented media is called *complete* or *growth media*. Complete media is typically used for basic cell culture maintenance and population expansion; it is also used as the positive control in most experiments due to its known impact on cells.

A basic cell experiment will include a negative and positive control, along with a range of treatment dosages. Each control and treatment group is set up with multiple replicates, referred to as the "n" value. For example, if you have n=5, then there are 5 individual test groups for each type of treatment. These replicates are compared to ensure credibility by running statistical tests during data analysis. If there is too large of variance within the replicates, data cannot be used.

A sample experiment including controls and treatments in a 96-well plate format may look like the following, in Figure 29.

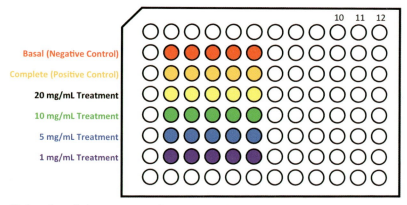

Basal (Negative Control)
Complete (Positive Control)
20 mg/mL Treatment
10 mg/mL Treatment
5 mg/mL Treatment
1 mg/mL Treatment

Figure 29. Sample study design in a 96-well plate layout, showing treatment and positive and negative control groups.

Note: A general rule for *in vitro* studies advises against plating cells in the outer boundary of an experimental plate due to a higher rate of media evaporation and varied cellular activity.

At the beginning of a cell based experiment, the cells must be seeded. *Cell seeding* simply means: to distribute a designated number or volume of cells over a given surface area. While cell stocks are typically grown in flasks, experimental designs usually require relocation of the cells to a culture plate. The plating density (number of cells per well) is determined based on the individual cell's growth requirements, cell size, and the length of study, which correlate with the number of cells that can fit in a given area and maintain viability or growth over the course of the experiment. *Confluence* is the term used to describe the proportion of surface area covered by adherent cells; for instance, a surface area with 50% confluence is half covered with cells. A 100% confluent cell monolayer can be seen in Figure 30.

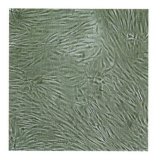

Figure 30. Example of cells in culture at 100% confluence.

There are two types of cells: cells which produce adherent proteins and will attach to a surface, and cells which remain suspended in their media. Adherent cell types require an enzyme called trypsin to gently remove cells from the surface of a flask for seeding. *Trypsin* is a digestive enzyme which degrades the attachment proteins of these cells from each other and the cell culture surface. This ability to chemically detach cells from a surface is valuable because manual removal can be very harsh and potentially damage cell membranes. Since trypsinization will cause the cells to round up and detach from a surface, adherent cells must be plated a day before treatment to allow for reattachment, membrane repair, and substrate spreading in their relaxed state.

As cell stocks cultured in flasks increase in number, they will also need to be trypsinized and subcultured into additional flasks for further growth expansion. The number of times a cell has been subcultured, or removed from its culture vessel, is called its *passage* number. Most normal cell types have a limited number of passages in which the cells can maintain their optimal, healthy characteristics in culture. Cells are typically passaged when their confluence reaches ~80% to prevent overcrowding issues which may affect growth rate or gene expression.

6.3 STANDARD CURVE

A *standard curve* is a graph that shows the relationship between two quantities; it is used to find the value of an unknown quantity based off of values given by known samples. This is performed by analyzing a number of known concentrations of material (for example, a known number of cells or amount of protein) to measure the outcome (such as absorbance or fluorescence) and create a linear relationship which can be determined mathematically.

For example, a known number of cells can be plated and quantified by various detection methods. The value assigned to each known number of cells will increase as the number of cells increases. By plotting a wide range of known values, unknown values may be extrapolated, as shown in Figure 31. Therefore, when the experimental sample is quantified, the value can be directly related to cell number using the standard curve.

Example:

Question:

Using the standard curve shown in Figure 31, if the experimental sample was quantified at a value of 157.21 units (y-axis), how many cells were in the sample (x-axis)?

Answer:

$y = 0.0196 * x + 0.41$

$x = (y - 0.41) / 0.0196$

$x = (157.21 - 0.41) / 0.0196$

$x = 8000$ cells

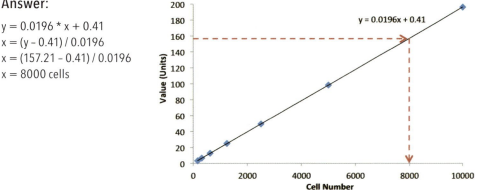

Figure 31. Example standard curve showing how an arbitrary outcome measure, such as absorbance or fluorescence, can be mathematically correlated to determine a numerical value of interest, such as cell number.

6.4 PLATE READER

A *plate reader* (or microplate reader) is an instrument used to quantify a biological, chemical, or physical event in multiple sample wells simultaneously. In other words, it is a method for quickly obtaining a value for a factor that cannot be counted by hand. These detections are made possible by adding a reagent to each sample well which binds only to the designated factor or event in question. Even though the same amount of reagent is added to each well, only the bound or activated reagent will be detectable by the plate reader. So if one is attempting to quantify the amount of VEGF in multiple sample wells, a VEGF binding reagent, such as a specific antibody, is added to each well but will only be detectible for the amount that VEGF is present in the sample. The reagent is measured through absorbance, fluorescence, or luminescence by the plate reader. These values require a standard curve to then be related back to the factor in question.

Absorbance: A laser is shined through the sample and the percent of light that is absorbed by the sample reagent is measured at a specified wavelength. Generally, the greater the amount of sample reagent present, the more light will be absorbed. Absorbance of light by a solution is correlated to transmission of light through a solution as measured by a detector, where %absorbance = 100% - %transmission.

Fluorescence: A laser illuminates (or excites) the sample reagent which, as a result, emits fluorescent light at a specified wavelength that is measured by the plate reader.

Luminescence: No laser is needed for this method, which uses biological or chemical reactions to create a detected photon measurement at a specified wavelength and is detected using a plate reader.

6.5 PREPARATION OF TISSUE EXTRACTS

For *in vitro* cell culture experiments, a tissue extract is a solution which contains soluble factors that are non-chemically released from a piece of tissue into the surrounding liquid. A single layer of cells *in vitro* is highly sensitive, and direct contact with solid components or tissue may physically disrupt the cell monolayer. Rather, a tissue extract is used as treatment to model the diffusion of the tissue's soluble factors to specific cell types in a wound.

Tissue extracts are prepared by finely mincing tissue to maximize surface area. These bits of tissue are then placed in the appropriate basal media for the specific cell type which is to be treated. All treatment extracts are prepped in basal media since it does not provide supplemented nourishment to the cells, and therefore cellular reactions can be regarded as the tissue extract's impact. If the extract was prepared in complete media, the benefits of the serum could mask the tissue's abilities. Once the minced tissue is in basal media, it is allowed to agitate overnight in a refrigerator to elute soluble components from the tissue and prevent protein degradation. Previous studies have shown that the maximum amounts of soluble components are released through this process after 24 hours. The extract is then sterile filtered in order to eliminate pieces of tissue and potential contaminants before treating cells.

Various concentrations of extract can be prepared by weighing the tissue and calculating the milligram of tissue to milliliter of media ratio. Once the extract is prepared, serial dilutions can be made by adding basal media to observe a wide range of responses, based on the relative concentrations of extract. For tissue extracts of MiMedx dHACM, cells are typically treated in the range of 20 mg/mL to 1 mg/mL, where the maximum impact is notable. Concentrations above 20 mg/mL may, in some cases, be too potent for *in vitro* studies as cells cultured in monolayer and not within 3D matrices may be more vulnerable to overstimulation, while below 1 mg/mL the impacts may be negligible.

6.6 CELL PROLIFERATION

Cell *proliferation* is the increase of cell number due to cell division. The cells used in wound studies replicate by a process called mitosis, where one cell divides to become two identical cells. Proliferation is the phase of wound healing following hemostasis and inflammation. During this phase the tissue is rebuilt through deposits of extracellular matrix (ECM) and collagen, in which blood vessel formation occurs.

The overall concept of a proliferation experiment is to compare the number of cells you have before and after treatment. The rate by which a population of cells doubles varies greatly based on cell type, cell donor, cell or donor age and health, and environmental stimuli. Typically MiMedx proliferation experiments span a 72 hour period. This period allows enough time to see statistical variance in cell numbers, while also ensuring that sufficient nutrients are available in one dosage of treatment.

There is a low initial seeding density for proliferation experiments to allow ample room for population growth. After adherent cells have attached overnight, all complete media is discarded and rinsed from the cells so as not to interfere with treatment. Basal media, complete media, and tissue extract dilutions are then individually added to the designated number of replicates and allowed to incubate with the cells for 72 hours. At the end of the experiment, all media is discarded and rinsed so that only healthy, attached cells remain.

An assay called a CyQuant (Life Technologies, Carlsbad, CA) can be used to gain a count of the final number of cells by DNA content in each well. A combination of lysis buffer and freezing the cells will cause the cells to *lyse*, or break down their membranes to expose DNA. The dye included in the CyQuant kit is then able to bind to the DNA of each individual cell. Once bound, the dye will fluoresce and a plate reader is used to quantify the fluorescence in each well. Since the quantification of DNA remains constant for each cell in a given cell type it can be used to calculate cell number by the generated standard curve.

6.7 CELL MIGRATION

Cell migration is the self-movement of cells from one location to another. Cells migrate in response to various factors including the need to feed, morphology developments, and environmental cues. Cell migration experiments represent a biological agent's ability to recruit cells in the body. There are multiple ways to look at migration of adherent cells *in vitro*; some evaluations simply identify a treatment's ability to promote general cell movement, while other studies can analyze migration in a specific direction.

An important factor for obtaining credible migration data is ensuring that proliferation does not interfere with the assay. Proliferation can exaggerate migration results if one cell migrates and then divides into multiple cells at its new location. To prevent this, cells are treated before the experiment with an agent called Mitomycin C. *Mitomycin C* (MMC) is a chemical that cross links the cell's DNA, thereby inhibiting nuclear division and eliminating proliferative abilities. This step is necessary for all *in vitro* studies solely focusing on migration.

6.7.1 CLOSURE ASSAYS

A general migration experiment will analyze cell movement in response to treatment without designated migration pathway. These assays are considered closure assays because cells plated around a void surface area may migrate to close the acellular gap. The percent closure of cells with high migratory activity in response to treatment will be much higher than of those cells treated with the negative control. This method of evaluation models the migration of surrounding cells into a ruptured cellular layer.

There are two formats commonly used for closure assays, as shown in Figure 32. In a scratch wound assay, a confluent layer of cells is manually scratched to disrupt one line of the confluent cell layer. In a wound closure assay, cells are plated surrounding a gel dot which dissolves in the media to leave a circular cell-free zone. Both assays allow the healthy surrounding cells to incubate directly in their treatments and potentially migrate into the acellular scratch or circular gap.

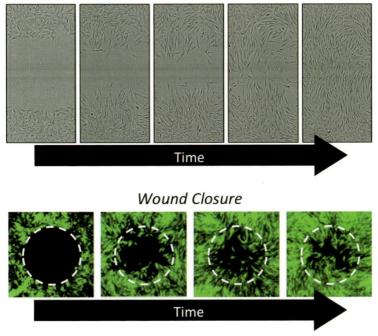

Figure 32. Scratch wound and wound closure migration assays. In a scratch wound (top panel; phase contrast) or wound closure (bottom panel; cells fluorescently labeled green) migration assay, cells migrate inward over time to fill an initially cell-free zone and rate of closure is measured.

6.7.2 CHEMOTAXIS ASSAYS

Directional migration studies are called chemotaxis assays. When a cell migrates toward or away from a chemical it is called *chemotaxis;* these signals which promote chemotaxis are called chemokines, as discussed previously. Therefore, these studies analyze a cell's migration toward a specific signal or treatment. To maximize this response, cells are serum and/or nutrient starved prior to analyzing their movement. This means that they are sustained by basal media for 24 hours rather than supplemented media, leaving them 'starving' for nourishment and chemotactic factors once they are plated. The goal of starving the cells is to maximize the cell's immediate response to treatment.

Chemotaxis assays are performed using transwell-plates which have one small, removable transwell microporous membrane inserted inside of a larger well. The starved cells are suspended in basal media very densely inside the transwell insert, and are then allowed to migrate through the permeable membrane toward the treatment below, as exemplified in Figure 33.

Transwell Chemotaxis Assay

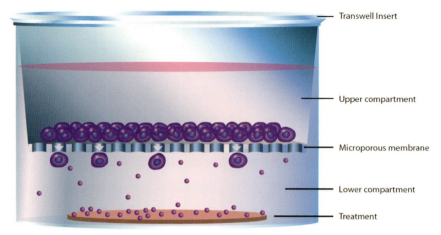

Transwell Insert

Upper compartment

Microporous membrane

Lower compartment

Treatment

Figure 33. Transwell chemotaxis assay.

It is crucial that there is no complete media added inside of the insert, which will counteract motivation for the cells to migrate toward the treatment. As soluble treatment signals prompt, the starved cells will migrate toward them through pores in the permeable membrane barrier. The permeable membrane supporting the cells has microscopic pores that can be designated for various sizes ranging from 0.4-12.0 micrometers. The pore size should be small enough so that cells are required to actively move themselves through the pore and will not simply fall through the membrane. After adherent cells migrate through the pores they adhere to the bottom surface of the membrane.

Transwell migration studies are typically limited to 24 hours once the cells are plated. By this point soluble components have diffused through the membrane and both the well and insert media are at equilibrium. Once equilibrium of the top and bottom media is reached, the cells no longer have directional motivation to migrate so the assay is complete. It is very important that negative and positive controls be included in the study. A positive control can be enriched culture medium or medium with specific chemotactic factors relevant to comparison with the test material added, while the negative control is often basal medium without any added chemotactic factors.

Serial dilutions of test materials can be placed in the lower wells in a basal media solution, or an agar gradient method can be used, in order to create a gradient of exposure and to maximize the time period before equilibrium. The agar gradient method is performed by embedding the treatment in *agarose gel*. Agarose is a polysaccharide extracted from seaweed which will go into solution when boiled, but will gel at room temperature. While in solution, agarose is mixed with the treatment and allowed to set as a gel. Basal media is then used to cover the gel so that soluble components will diffuse slowly into the media, forming a diffusion gradient to the cells suspended above.

Following the 24 hour experimental period, the numbers of cells which have migrated through the pores and attached to the bottom surface of the membrane are analyzed. This is done by various methods of either staining and counting the attached cells or by enzymatically detaching cells from the surface with a dissociation solution such as trypsin. Use of CyQuant dye in combination with a high concentration of lysis buffer will allow the detached cells to be fluorescently dyed and evaluated by the plate reader. Alternatively, the cells can be labeled with a fluorescent dye, and then evaluated for transwell migration of the cells to the bottom surface of the membranes using a fluorescent plate reader or microscope.

6.8 GROWTH FACTOR, CYTOKINE AND CHEMOKINE MEASUREMENTS

The majority of growth factor, cytokine and chemokine quantitative assays are based upon the Enzyme-Linked Immunosorbent Assay (ELISA) methodology. The ELISA uses the innate specificity of antibodies to antigens to accurately determine the concentration of a molecule of interest, known as an antigen, from a complex sample. Depending on the assay, the signal can be read using absorbance, fluorescence or luminescence. Within the ELISA methodology, there are many variations including: sandwich ELISA, direct ELISA, competitive ELISA and more. The ELISA platform has also been multiplexed to make the assay more high-throughput for screening large numbers of growth factors. An example of this type of ELISA application is the Quantibody array (Raybiotech, Norcoss, GA).

The sandwich ELISA is the most common and usually the most sensitive of all the ELISA assays. Also, it is the principle employed in the multiplexed Quantibody array; therefore, the mechanism by which is works will be elaborated.

The sandwich ELISA measures the amount of antigen between two layers of antibodies (capture and detection)—hence the moniker 'sandwich' ELISA. In brief, samples are applied to a plate coated with a primary antibody, specific to the antigen or molecule of interest. The specificity of the primary antibody, coated on the plate, prevents non-specific binding; therefore, only the antigen is detected in the test sample. Unbound sample is washed away and a secondary antibody, conjugated to a reporter enzyme or fluorophore, binds a different region of the antigen, captured by the primary antibody. Unbound secondary antibody complex is washed away and an enzyme substrate is added and cleaved by the bound enzyme on the secondary antibody. The resultant signal produced is proportional to the concentration of the molecule of interest based on a standard curve of known antigen concentrations that is compared to the test sample readings to define the concentrations of antigen in the test samples.

6.9 HISTOLOGICAL STAINING

Histological staining, including special stains, immunohistochemistry, and immunocytochemistry, can provide valuable visual information by labeling specific structures, cell markers, or markers of viability in tissues and cell cultures. Typically, tissues are embedded in an embedding medium, either frozen in OCT (Optimal Cutting Temperature) compound or in paraffin wax, allowing them to be sectioned into very thin, 5 μm thick cross-sectional slices, as depicted in Figure 34.

Cross-Sectional Tissue Section

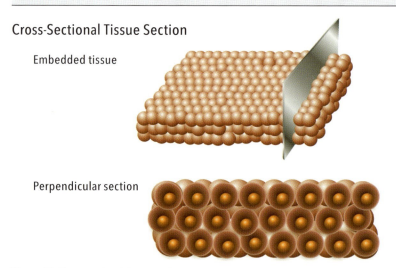

Embedded tissue

Perpendicular section

Figure 34. Cross-sectional tissue section.

These thin tissue sections mounted on slides, as well as cultured cells, can then be stained and labeled with specific markers. Common stains include hematoxylin and eosin (H&E) for cell nuclei, Alcian blue for acidic polysaccharides/proteoglycans, Masson's trichrome for collagen, and Verhoeff's stain for elastic fibers. H&E stains cell nuclei dark blue with hematoxylin, while cell cytoplasm and extracellular matrix are counterstained pink with eosin. Alcian blue stains glycosaminoglycans and proteoglycans blue, and cell nuclei are counterstained red with nuclear red stain. Masson's trichrome stains collagen blue, cell cytoplasm red, and cell nuclei black. Verhoeff's stains elastic fibers black, and collagen matrix pink with Van Gieson's stain.

Additionally, similar to ELISA, the innate specificity of antibodies can be used to label cellular and matrix component through immunohistochemistry and immunocytochemistry. First, a primary antibody which specifically binds to the antigen of interest is used to detect the molecule of interest, as shown in Figure 35. For example, a mouse anti-human collagen Type I antibody is an antibody raised in mice that specifically binds to human collagen Type I. Then, a secondary antibody which is labelled with a special tag and specifically binds the primary antibody can be used to detect the presence or absence of antigen. For example, a goat anti-mouse IgG antibody is raised in a goat to specifically bind mouse IgG type antibodies. The secondary antibodies are conjugated with reactive enzymes (such as alkaline phosphatase or horseradish peroxidase that react with color changing substrates) or fluorescent fluorophores (of any color) to then visualize the presence of the antibody complex and indirectly the antigen under a microscope.

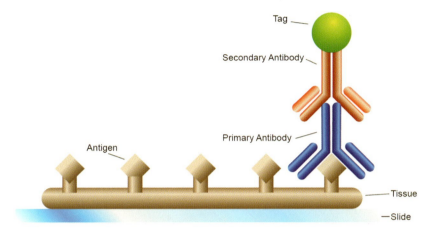

Figure 35. Immunostaining using labeled antibodies.

Additional stains can use other aspects of cell activity and structure to demonstrate cellular characteristics. For example, LIVE/DEAD stain uses calcein to stain live cells to fluoresce green and ethidium homodimer-1 to stain dead cells to fluoresce red. In this stain, calcein is cell permeable and is cleaved within the cytosol of viable and metabolically active cells by intracellular esterase activity to fluoresce green. Ethidium homodimer-1, however, is not membrane permeable but can enter the ruptured cell membranes of nonviable cells, binding nuclear DNA and fluorescing red.

6.10 GENE EXPRESSION

Reverse transcription polymerase chain reaction (RT-PCR) is an experimental technique used to determine gene expression of a group of cells. Genes in the form of DNA are expressed through mRNA signals which are then translated into protein; therefore, mRNA is a direct reflection of gene expression. Using RT-PCR, mRNA is reverse transcribed (RT) back into a form a DNA called complementary DNA (cDNA), and then polymerase chain reaction (PCR) is used to exponentially replicate cDNA for quantification. This technique is performed using thermally stable enzymes that copy DNA from a template strand. mRNA is reverse transcribed into cDNA using reverse transcriptase enzyme. Then the cDNA is replicated using a series of thermocycles (cycles of heating and cooling) with Taq DNA polymerase enzyme which is thermally stable up to 95°C. Taq polymerase was originally isolated from *Thermus aquaticus* bacterium, which thrives in elevated temperatures of hot springs and hydrothermal vents; therefore, Taq polymerase can withstand and remain activate at elevated temperature where human enzymes cannot.

In the first step of PCR, the sample is heated to 95°C causing the strands of the DNA double helix to denature or separate into single strands, as depicted in Figure 36. After this, the sample is cooled to 50°C, where short DNA primers that define a sequence of interest bind to the cDNA strands. These primers are designed to flank a cDNA region specific to the gene of interest. For example, if the mRNA sequence that corresponds

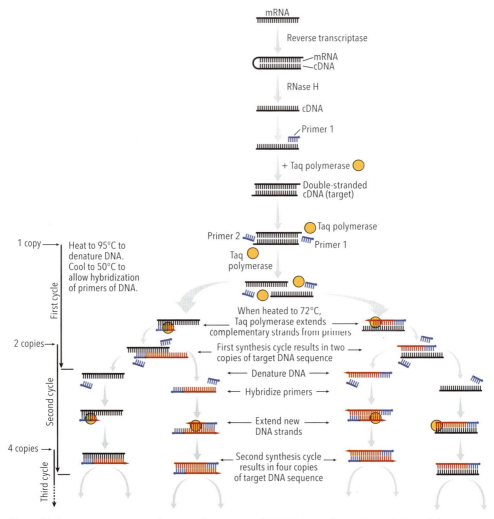

Figure 36. Reverse transcription polymerase chain reaction (RT-PCR) transcribes mRNA to cDNA, and then uses sequence specific primers to replicate cDNA for quantification.

to collagen Type I gene expression is known, then two primers (one sequence for each cDNA strand) can be designed that would only bind and replicate genes representing collagen Type I. Following primer annealing, the sample is then heated to 72°C where Taq polymerase is active and copies the DNA strands. These three temperature stages represent a single thermocycle, and in each cycle the cDNA of interest doubles in number. A single gene becomes 2 copies, then 4 copies, then 8, etc. By increasing exponentially, a single gene can be amplified 2^{40} or 1,099,511,627,776 times in 40 thermocycles.

In quantitative PCR, fluorescent probes are used to quantify cDNA content, correlating back to the starting content of cDNA. As the thermocycles progress, the cDNA replicates resulting in an increase in fluorescence as shown in Figure 37. Therefore, gene targets with higher gene expression are amplified at earlier cycle numbers than gene targets with lower expression, which are expressed later.

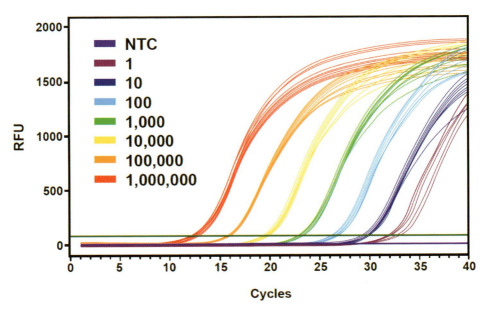

Figure 37. Fluorescence vs. thermocycles quantitative PCR plot. The PCR amplification curves demonstrate how gene targets with higher gene expression (red: 1,000,000) are amplified at earlier cycle numbers than gene targets with lower expression (maroon: 1), which are expressed later.

CHAPTER 7

IN VIVO ANIMAL MODELS

Similar to the *in vitro* models described in Chapter 6, MiMedx also utilizes *in vivo* animal studies as model systems to analyze the biological properties of PURION Processed dHACM products. The importance of well-controlled preclinical models, as well as a description of the models used by MiMedx are discussed here in Chapter 7.

7.1 USE OF PRECLINICAL MODELS

Rodent models have been extensively utilized for many of MiMedx's preclinical assessments of dHACM safety and mechanism of action for soft tissue healing. Use of rodents is advantageous for a number of reasons: (a) they represent a dynamic, mammalian *in vivo* (Latin for "within the living") system; (b) they have been used extensively in preclinical testing; (c) results from mammalian animals can be more readily extrapolated to humans than *in vitro* laboratory bench-top or biochemical testing; (d) appropriate numbers of replicates can be used to better ensure power of statistical analyses, proper interpretation of study results, and the ability to draw conclusions to evaluate medical products; and (e) their housing and care are relatively inexpensive. There are also a broad range of surgical models available in rodents for testing medical products and surgery does not require sophisticated surgical facilities other than providing a sterile field in a relatively small space.

Disadvantages of rodent models include that they are small, accompanied by smaller organs and tissues, are more distantly related phylogenetically to humans than other species (for example, non-human primates), and they respond with a very robust healing response to most injuries. The latter characteristic can make it difficult to observe improvement in healing outcomes in rodents following treatment of a wound, for example, with a medical product when compared to untreated (sham) control wounds. However, despite the fact that all animal models have benefits and drawbacks, we can learn much about the basic biological characteristics of a medical product from animal studies. Today they continue to be used to establish preclinical toxicity, pharmacology, pharmacokinetics, toxicokinetics, and biodistribution of medical substances, devices, and biomaterials destined for use as clinical treatments for medical needs in humans. In fact, animal study data remains a cornerstone of the Food and Drug Administration (FDA) for regulatory submissions to assess safety and efficacy and gain approval for the initiation of human clinical trials and ultimately approval to commercialize medical products.

Preclinical studies in animals are a common element of drug, biologic, and medical device development. *In vitro* (translated directly from the Latin, "in glass," generally refers to experiments conducted in a laboratory or outside of the body) laboratory bench-top models provide good preliminary scientific evidence for the evaluation of a product's mechanism of action. However, *in vitro* cell culture models are tested in a two-dimensional environment that does not replicate the complex, three-dimensional tissue architecture and environments that cells encounter in the body. In addition, *in vitro* models represent "static" or closed systems where there is generally limited or no fluid exchange. The latter tends to result in cumulative, long-term exposure of responder cells in culture to any reagents or biological factors released from the test product that stimulates a response from the cells (e.g., proliferation or migration).

In vivo animal models represent a platform for evaluating the safety and mechanism of action of a medical product in a dynamic, three-dimensional, living environment. While animals and humans differ in many respects, they are similar in that the complex interactions among ECM, cells, blood flow, a functioning immune system, nervous system, and other essential organ systems are in play and operational for evaluating the properties of a drug or biologic. For a product like dHACM, animal models provide an opportunity to learn more about its mechanism of action in healing different tissues, its safety, and the amount of time the body requires to break down and incorporate the product (bioresorption). *In vitro* testing has not yet been scientifically validated, or in many cases, is simply not yet available as an option to provide data in these areas of interest related to medical product evaluation prior to testing the product in humans in clinical trials. FDA recommends that all *in vivo* and *in vitro* preclinical safety testing be performed in compliance with a set of guidelines known as Good Laboratory Practices, or GLP, which is described in the Code of Federal Regulations, in a section called "21 CFR, part 58."

Animal models may be limited as to the extent to which the responses to a medical product observed in the animals can be extrapolated to humans. Differences in biological responses to medical products are known to exist between animals and humans. One example of this is the fact that animals tend to heal more rapidly and robustly than humans do, and that they do not develop chronic conditions, such as chronic wounds, the way humans often do. Thus, it can be challenging to demonstrate the efficacy of a product in animals because they do not develop chronically, stalled healing responses the way humans do, even following induction of disease states in the animals, such as diabetes. Another example is that animals, particularly rodents, may clear administered drugs more rapidly from their bodies than humans are likely to do, reducing the time for interaction of the drug with the tissues and organs of the animal compared to what would be experienced in humans. This is not always true for every medical product, but it is necessary to temper interpretation of outcomes observed in animal subjects with these potential shortcomings in mind, and why it is critical to perform clinical trials to validate the safety and efficacy of medical products in human subjects.

The design of animal studies to include positive and negative controls against which to compare test materials is important. As with any other type of scientific experiment, from *in vitro* laboratory, in vivo preclinical to human clinical trials, the principles of good scientific method apply to better ensure generation of experimental data that can be readily interpreted, and to allow the investigator to draw conclusions that increase our understanding of a product being tested. Inclusion of well-conceived controls and enough replicates in each test and control group included in the study design to overcome any inherent natural variability in the model chosen as a testing platform is critical to success. Animal studies are often designed so that every animal in the study includes an "internal, sham" control. In a dermal wound study, for example, what this means is that in addition to wounds on each animal that received treatment with a test product, another wound be included on each animal that received no test product, which would act as a sham surgical control to compare against the wounds that received test product. The word "internal" control is also used to describe this type of control, because it is included in the same animal as the testing sites to allow direct comparisons. Including internal, sham controls in each animal also helps to compensate for inherent, animal-to-animal variability, allowing the investigator to observe an effect due to a test product if one were to exist, and reducing the number of animals needed for inclusion in the overall study design. One potential drawback to a design of this sort is that the test product can elicit a far-reaching "systemic" effect in the test animals and influence the outcome at the control site. An example of a systemic effect would be if a drug administered at one site on the body traveled through the blood to influence another site on the animal's body remote from where the drug was initially administered. Illustration of test product treatment sites and internal, sham control sites in the same animal is shown in Figure 38. In the case of dHACM, the effects that have been observed in human and animal studies so far, suggests that its effects are localized to the site of application for accelerating healing, and that systemic effects at remote sites in the same person or animal subject are unlikely to occur.

It is also acceptable to include separate groups of control animals in an animal study design. This requires the inclusion of larger numbers of animals in the study, but has the benefit of providing test and control data where the outputs from one or the other treatment cannot unexpectedly influence the other. This type of design is common for evaluating the toxicology of test products, where it is desired to understand the overall impact of treating a test animal with a medical product in isolation, and compare it against animals that have undergone the same surgical procedure, but which did not receive the test product treatment in question.

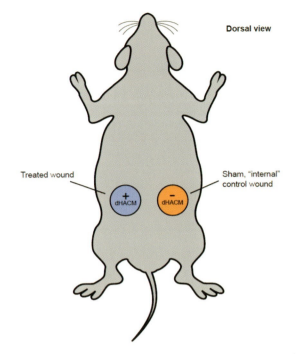

Figure 38. Schematic illustration of a rodent with test article treatment and a sham control. The "back" (dorsal) aspect of an animal subject contains two wounds: one of which receives treatment with a test product (blue), and another that receives no treatment to act as a "sham, internal" negative control (orange). This is a common animal study design feature for test products expected to have a localized effect at the site of treatment to improve understanding of the product's efficacy and mechanism of action compared to a control site in the same animal.

For both types of study designs it is necessary to include an appropriate number of animals per test and control group to ensure one can draw conclusions based on the data from the study. This is accomplished using a statistical approach known as "power analysis," which takes into account the expected level of variability in the primary outcome one wishes to learn more about with regard to the test product being evaluated. The expected variability in the outcome of interest can be ascertained from similar studies that were previously performed and reported in the scientific literature by other investigators, or from data generated from previous studies conducted in-house using the same animal model.

The following is an arbitrary example using percentage of wound closure data in an animal model of dermal wound healing. If the wound closure observed in an animal model after 7 days with treatment was on *average* 40% with a *standard deviation* of 10%, then the percent variance in that data was *standard deviation* divided by *average* and multiplied by 100 or in this case, (10 divided by 40)*100 = 25%. Thus, the results from this previous study indicated that we could expect 25% variance in the wound closure outcomes in this animal model. The percent variance is also known as a "coefficient of variation" and can be used in conjunction with statistical analysis software to conduct a power analysis to predict how many animals per group will be needed to increase the chances (typically set at a value of 80% probability) of observing a statistically significant difference between treated and control wounds for wound closure at any given timepoint in a future study. With this approach, statistical relevance can be achieved.

7.2 DETAILS OF ANIMAL MODELS USED

To date, MiMedx has published several peer-reviewed scientific manuscripts describing the results of preclinical evaluations of dHACM in various rodent animal models.[73-75,77,104] All studies conducted by MiMedx were conducted according to a study protocol which is rigorously reviewed and approved both internally and independently by the external testing site's Institutional Animal Care and Use Committee (IACUC) to ensure that the study procedures are ethical, will not lead to unnecessary distress or discomfort to the animals, and cannot be reproduced using *in vitro* model systems in the laboratory. The company designs animal studies with the principle of the 3 "R's" in mind which include reducing the number of animals used for testing, refining models to minimize animal discomfort and suffering and improving animal welfare, and replacing animal testing wherever possible. MiMedx works with testing sites that operate in compliance with international regulations for animal care established by the National Institutes of Health (NIH) and the Association for Assessment and Accreditation of Laboratory Animal Care (AAALAC).

7.2.1 MESENCHYMAL STEM CELL (MSC) RECRUITMENT

The first data suggesting that implantation of dHACM *in vivo* leads to the recruitment of host mesenchymal stem cells was published in Koob, T.J., et al. (2013).[73] A mouse model was used in which an ischemic skin flap is created by a surgical incision to separate a flap of the epidermis layer of skin from the underlying dermis. This has the effect of reducing the blood supply to the epidermal skin flap, creating conditions of "ischemia" which essentially means there is a restriction in blood supply to the skin flap. This model was used to simulate the poor blood supply to chronic wounds such as diabetic foot ulcers (DFUs). An illustration is provided in Figure 39, showing how the ischemic flap mouse model was used to evaluate dHACM for stem cell recruitment in the publication.[73] An important feature to note is the inclusion of two types of negative controls in each animal. The first control is called a "sham" surgical control in which a surgical ischemic flap site is created but receives no treatment. In general, sham control sites are included for comparison to "test" sites that receive treatment. Often, sham sites are included in the same animal as the "test" site to account for baseline levels of the biological responses being measured, and to account for variability in response from animal to animal.

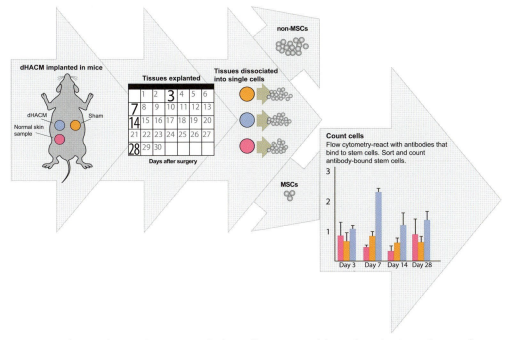

Figure 39. Schematic diagram depicting use of ischemic flap mouse model to evaluate dHACM implantation for the recruitment of stem cells. Stem cell recruitment was compared to a "sham" surgical control and to normal, uninjured skin in each animal.[73]

In this instance, after euthanizing animals on various days after surgery, the wound site tissues were harvested and enzymatically dissociated to yield the single cells that make part of the tissue. The enzyme used to do this is called "collagenase," and is active in degrading all of the collagen matrix surrounding the cells in the tissue, releasing them to yield a suspension of single cells. The single cells are then exposed to antibodies bound to molecules that fluoresce in different colors depending on which site on the cell they bind to specifically. Those cells that are bound by a particular antibody can be "sorted" based on the fluorescence molecule they are tagged with, using a device called a flow cytometer. The flow cytometer not only sorts the cells, but can also count the cells that are tagged with a particular antibody. In this instance, cells that did not bind to an antibody for a cell-surface protein marker, called CD45, i.e., CD45- cells, but which did bind to an antibody for another cell-surface protein marker, called Sca-1, i.e., Sca-1+ cells, were considered to be MSCs and were counted among the single cell suspensions yielded from each wound site. As shown in the diagram above, there were more CD45-/Sca-1+ MSCs counted among the cells present at wound sites treated with PURION Processed dHACM after 7 days post-treatment than in sham control or normal skin control tissues. The data provided evidence that PURION Processed dHACM implanted in ischemic wound sites leads to enhanced stem cell recruitment into the implantation site.

7.2.2 HEMATOPOIETIC STEM CELL (HSC) RECRUITMENT

A second study was conducted in mice, with the exception that the surgical model used was one in which dHACM and a control acellular fetal bovine dermal matrix (ADM, PriMatrix, TEI Biosciences) were implanted into individual subcutaneous pockets created on the flanks of each of the animals.[77] From a surgical perspective, subcutaneous pockets differ from ischemic skin flaps in that they simply involve an incision through the skin down to the muscle fascia layer of tissue, and generally do not result in a restriction of blood supply to the surgical site. A test sample, such as dHACM, was inserted into the subcutaneous pocket and then the tissues are closed in layers with sutures over the implant. Subcutaneous sites treated with dHACM, ADM, or that received no experimental treatment to act as sham surgical control sites were harvested at 3, 7, 14, and 28 days after surgery. The harvested tissues were dissected into halves, and one half was processed for histological sectioning and immunohistochemical staining for the hematopoietic progenitor cell (HPC)-surface marker CD34 to identify and quantify HPCs present in the tissues. Immunohistochemistry is a technique used to specifically stain molecular biomarkers using antibody reagents on histological tissue sections mounted on a microscope slide, and the process is shown schematically in Figure 40.

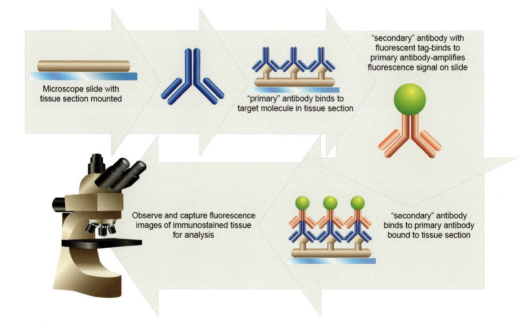

Figure 40. Diagram illustrating process of staining tissue sections mounted on microscope slides for molecular biomarkers by indirect immunofluorescence. Images not shown to scale.

For the purposes of this Primer, the antibody CD34 is predominantly expressed on the surface of HPCs, so it serves as a good marker to identify these cells in tissue sections. CD34$^+$ HPCs in the tissue sections were quantified by microscopic image analysis and compared among the different treatments and controls at each timepoint. Quantities of CD34$^+$ HPCs were statistically significantly higher both in tissues surrounding PURION Processed dHACM ("peri-implant") and within the dHACM implant material itself ("intra-implant") 14 and 28 days after surgery, compared to sites implanted with ADM, sham control sites and normal, healthy skin tissue. These data provided preclinical evidence *in vivo* that PURION Processed dHACM implantation stimulates enhanced recruitment of hematopoietic stem cells to the implanted tissues.

The other half of each tissue from the same study was dissociated into a single cell suspension using the enzyme collagenase, and the cells were subjected to separation by flow cytometry to quantify the HPCs present.[77] This method again involved treating the dissociated cell suspensions with a cocktail of antibodies specific for cell-surface markers present on HPCs. The cell-surface markers in this case consisted of CD45, c-Kit, and Sca-1. CD45 is a cell-surface receptor/enzyme complex found on all hematopoietic cells. c-Kit is a cell-surface protein receptor that binds to a cytokine molecule called, stem cell factor (SCF), and is expressed on bone marrow-derived HPCs. Sca-1, or stem cell antigen-1, is also expressed on the surface of HPCs. The antibodies in the cocktail that bind to these molecular cell-surface targets on HPCs were chemically bound to molecular tags that fluoresce at different wavelengths (different colors). Cells bound by all of the antibodies in the cocktail were defined as HPCs (i.e., they were CD45+/c-Kit+/Sca-1+), were sorted using a flow cytometer, and separated from cells that were negative for any of these markers (non-HPCs). In addition to separating the antibody-labeled HPCs from other cell types, the flow cytometer was used to count the number of HPCs isolated from each of the dissociated tissues recovered from the mice. Similarly to the results obtained by immunohistochemical staining of the tissues for HPCs, the flow cytometry also showed enhanced recruitment of HPCs to tissues implanted with PURION Processed dHACM 14 and 28 days after surgery, compared to ADM or control tissues. These data corroborated the immunohistochemistry findings that PURION Processed dHACM implantation leads to recruitment of HPCs to implant sites.

7.2.3 NEOVASCULARIZATION

A third study using the mouse ischemic flap surgical model was conducted, and was used to evaluate neovascularization of wound tissues implanted with dHACM.[75] Neovascularization is the formation of functional new capillary networks that carry red blood cells to tissues following an injury and is an essential biological process required for healing to occur. Similarly to the first study, ischemic wound flaps were surgically created on the backs (dorsal side) of mice, and then one wound was treated with dHACM, and the other was left untreated to act as a sham surgical control for comparison in each animal. A diagram of the experimental design is shown in Figure 41.

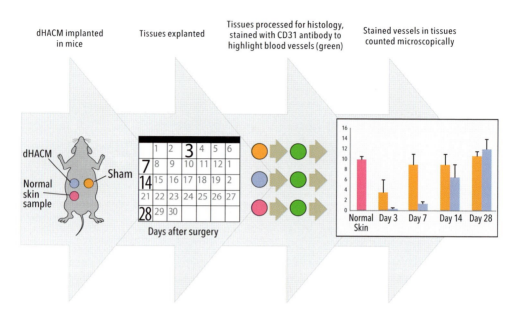

Figure 41. Schematic diagram depicting use of ischemic flap mouse model to evaluate dHACM implantation for neovascularization of wound tissues. Blood vessel counts were compared to "sham" surgical control ("injured skin") and to normal, uninjured skin in each animal. After 28 days, dHACM supported intra-implant neovascularization with an increase in the number of vessels within the dHACM grafts themselves to levels similar to normal and healing skin. Abbreviations: HPF = high-powered microscopic field of view.[75]

On each timepoint of the study, animals were euthanized and wound tissues were harvested and processed for histological sectioning. Thin sections through the wound tissues were stained by immunohistochemistry methods specifically to highlight new blood vessels. An antibody that binds to an endothelial cell-surface marker called CD31 that is chemically bound to a fluorescent molecule, was used to stain the new blood vessels in the tissue sections so that they glow green under a fluorescence microscope. The immunohistochemically stained $CD31^+$ vessels were counted in each tissue section under the microscope, to compare the number of blood vessels in treated, sham injured skin or normal skin samples. Recall that human amniotic membrane is "avascular," lacking any blood vessels, so the importance of the data shown is that the wounds treated with PURION Processed dHACM, which starts out having no blood vessels, become vascularized over the 28 days of the study eventually catching up with normal skin tissues, which in the mice were well-vascularized to begin with. The results of this second animal study demonstrated that PURION Processed dHACM stimulates angiogenesis in an in vivo ischemic wound animal model.

7.2.4 PARABIOSIS MODEL OF STEM CELL RECRUITMENT

A fourth study was conducted to further expand upon the understanding of how PURION Processed dHACM recruits host stem cells *in vivo*. This study again utilized the ischemic flap wound model in mice, but included an additional element of complexity and sophistication that enabled tracking and visualization of the stem cells' location and distribution in the tissues of the mice.[77] The model used has been described as the "green" mouse model, because one of a pair of mice used to generate the model system, was genetically altered such that every cell of its body expressed a fluorescent protein called green fluorescent protein (GFP). This "green" mouse was surgically connected by a flap of the dorsal skin to a dorsal skin flap of another mouse which was genetically identical other than not expressing GFP, so that its cells could not glow green. Two weeks after the surgery to connect the two mice, the animals shared their blood circulation (known as "parabiosis") such that blood and other cells, including circulating stem cells, from each animal flowed into the other through the blood circulation. The experimental design using this model to evaluate dHACM is illustrated in Figure 42.

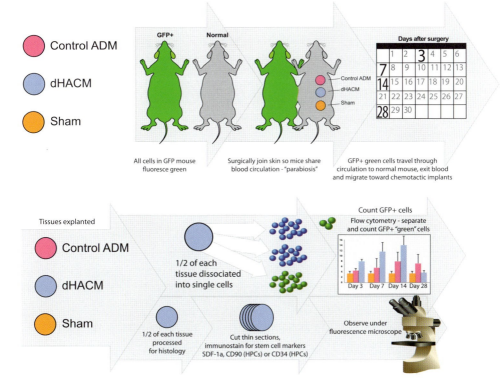

Figure 42. Flowchart showing surgical creation of "parabiosed" GFP+ mouse with normal mouse. Immunohistochemical and flow cytometry data were used to evaluate dHACM for recruitment of circulating HPCs.[77]

The flanks of each normal mouse (i.e., GFP⁻) in the pairing received subcutaneous implants of dHACM (EpiFix), ADM, or no experimental treatment to act as sham surgical controls under an ischemic flap of skin. As with a previously described study, the implant and control tissues were harvested at 3, 7, 14 and 28 days and divided in half for either immunohistochemical analysis or for dissociation into single cells for flow cytometry analysis. Recall that the key aspect of this study was that a GFP⁺ mouse was parabiosed with a normal GFP⁻ mouse, such that each pair of animals shared their blood circulation meaning that cells from each animal could travel in the blood into the other. Flow cytometry was used to show that GFP⁺ cells, i.e., "green" cells from the "green" mouse, were recruited to dHACM implant sites in the normal mouse. There was enhanced recruitment of GFP⁺ cells to PURION Processed dHACM implant sites compared with ADM sites or sham controls, suggesting that cells from the "green" mouse could travel through the circulation, and respond to signals released from dHACM by extruding from the blood vessels, and migrating into tissues in the normal mouse treated with PURION Processed dHACM more so than other treatments and controls.

Immunohistochemical staining of the remaining half of each implant site provided additional understanding of the GFP⁺ cells recruited from the circulation to the dHACM implant sites in the normal mice. Staining of tissue sections was conducted to detect a chemokine molecule known as stromal-derived factor-1alpha (SDF-1α), and is strongly chemotactic (i.e., it induces cells to migrate toward it) for hematopoietic cells including HPCs. An antibody that specifically binds to SDF-1α in tissue sections was used to fluorescently stain for the molecule. Images of the stained sections showed red fluorescent regions where SDF-1α was present, and separate images in the green fluorescent wavelength were taken of the same tissue to show where the GFP⁺ "green" cells were located. The two images were merged, or overlaid so that they lined up perfectly using image analysis software as shown in Figure 43, and the red (SDF-1α stained regions) and green fluorescent regions (GFP⁺ cells) were combined into one image. When GFP⁺ cells overlapped with SDF-1α⁺ regions, the combined result in the merged image is yellow-orange stained regions (red combined with green = orange), which indicate that SDF-1α and GFP are co-expressed in the same area of the image by the same cells. Increased SDF-1α detection in PURION Processed dHACM treated tissues, suggested a possible mechanism for the recruitment of the HPCs to the treated tissues.

Additional immunohistochemical staining of the tissues was performed to help positively identify HPCs in tissues treated with dHACM. Co-expression of an HPC cell-surface protein marker, CD90, and GFP was evaluated by immunohistochemistry and merging of images to overlay red (CD90) and green fluorescent (GFP) stained regions. The immunohistochemistry data for dHACM-treated tissues showed that CD90 and GFP were co-expressed further suggesting that circulating HPCs were recruited to tissues implanted with PURION Processed dHACM.

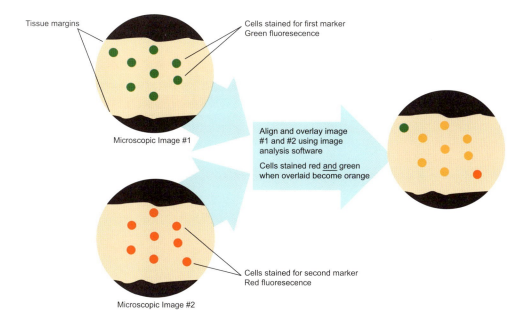

Figure 43. Overlaying immunofluorescent microscopic images to show co-expression of two different cellular biomarker molecules.

Finally, immunohistochemical staining of the new blood vessel biomarker, CD31 (red fluorescence), and detection of GFP$^+$ cells (green fluorescence) in dHACM-treated tissue sections showed some GFP$^+$ cells co-expressing CD31 (orange in merged images; red + green = orange on the color wheel) in and around blood vessel structures in the tissues. These results suggested that circulating GFP$^+$ cells colocalized with areas of neovascularization, and further suggesting that the recruited GFP$^+$ cells played a provascular role in-line with scientific literature reports that HPCs have angiogenic potential.

The results described from these preclinical rodent models are important indicators that PURION Processed dHACM affects biological systems in a variety of ways following surgical implantation *in vivo*. PURION Processed dHACM was demonstrated to recruit mesenchymal stem cells and hematopoietic stem cells from the blood circulation to the site of implantation, stimulate neovascularization at the site of implantation, and upregulate SDF-1α at the site of implantation. These biological responses all play important roles in the regulation of healing and repair within the human body, suggesting that clinically observed wounds may respond similarly following implantation of PURION Processed dHACM. These studies only used PURION Processed dHACM; therefore, the results of these studies do not apply to other tissue allografts. In fact, PURION Processed dHACM was shown to stimulate and recruit greater levels of stem cell migration when compared to a particular form of acellular dermal matrix (PriMatrix), processed by TEI Biosciences.

CHAPTER 8

CLINICAL TRIALS

8.1 INTRODUCTION

Clinical trials are medically based experiments undertaken on human subjects to systematically determine the effectiveness and/or safety of therapeutic interventions. Formal definitions of clinical trials are numerous, but they capture the concept of an organized, systematic study of human subjects in a treatment environment that is consistent.[245] Studies are created to measure different things, such as determining whether a treatment is effective compared to a placebo or determining whether one treatment is more effective than another. Increasingly, the cost of therapy is also being added into the studies to create what are called *cost effectiveness analyses*, in which the effectiveness of various therapies is being balanced against current treatments, delivery costs, and potential short and long-term outcomes related to overall patient care costs.

8.1.1 HISTORY

Clinical trials are part of a more broadly defined group of investigations that involve human subjects. Much of what constitutes the generally recognized appropriate behavior and ethics of researchers has evolved over the last century. In part, this process was accelerated by the medical experimentation that occurred in Germany during World War II and in other totalitarian regimes, and consensus on what constitutes correct conduct and performance of research has been codified on an international level and adopted and modified nationally in the United States. Several well-known documents have been developed to outline these principles including:

- The *Nuremburg Code of 1947* developed in response to the Nuremburg war trials.
- The *Helsinki Declaration of 1964*.
- The *1971 Guidelines by the US Department of Health Education and Welfare*, codified into formal Federal regulations in 1974.
- The *Belmont Report*, published in 1979 by the National Commission for the Protection of Human Subjects in Biomedical and Behavioral Research is

required reading for all researchers. This document provides the ethical underpinnings of most of the U.S. Federal regulations governing human research. The document sets out the difference between the practice of medicine and research, ethical principles including the principles of respect for individuals, beneficence and justice, and more specific the application of these principles to actual research. For example, the document discusses informed consent, the assessment of risks and benefits and the design of research, and the selection of subjects.

- The *International Conference on the Harmonization of Technical Requirements for the Registration of Pharmaceuticals for Human Use* guidance documents. Referred to usually as the *International Conference on Harmonization*, or ICH, this group developed international standards in the early 1990s that were adopted in large measure by the United States and once followed, permit the exportation of research results across international borders without the need for repetition or replication of studies.[246] An example is **ICH E6**, a standard that addresses how clinical trials are designed, executed and reported. The ICH group further developed the definitions of *Good Clinical Practice (GCP)* that form the basis of much of what is now standard practice in clinical research.

The manner in which clinical research is being conducted has been changing rapidly over the past decade. Governmental control and regulation has been steadily increasing. What previously had been identified as the **practice of medicine** (a formal research term used to distinguish physician practice evaluations) where physicians could undertake small scale internal studies in their practice, or where hospitals might do "continuous quality improvement" initiatives, increasing regulatory scrutiny has reshaped these processes.

While graduate level courses are taught on how to do clinical studies and entire books are written on this subject, there are some basic considerations that guide all of the basic research undertaken today. Clinicians and non-clinicians alike who supervise clinical studies must all be formally trained in the history and ethics of clinical trials and they must have GCP training.

8.1.2 REGULATORY ENVIRONMENT

The regulatory environment in which clinical trials are conducted must be considered by investigators under penalty from violating federal standards and laws. Information on what constitutes human research and how it must be conducted is clearly outlined by the Office for Human Research Protection (OHRP) and ClinicalTrials.gov on their websites.[247,248]

Clinical research in the USA is conducted under the auspices or under the direction of the FDA and its Centers: Center for Biologics Evaluation and Research (CBER), Center for Drug Evaluation and Research (CDER), and Center for Devices and Radiological Health (CDRH). Clinical research in the US must follow FDA guidelines and most of the ICH guidelines, and it must also be compliant with a large number of regulations and guidance documents specific to the field of investigation. International studies must follow intra-country and regional (e.g., European Union; EU) guidances, as well as FDA regulations if US-based institutions are involved or if the data will be used for the US market. Formal regulations define certain types of products and areas for intense review, based on the estimated risk involved and historic positioning by the FDA administrators.

Table IX. FDA classification of human tissue based medical products.

CLASSIFICATION	MARKETING PATHWAY	DESCRIPTION OF REQUIREMENTS
Section 361 HCT/Ps (human cells, tissues, and cellular and tissue-based products)	FDA clearance or approval not required	Minimally manipulated, intended for homologous use. No clearance or premarket approval required. Requires FDA current Good Tissue Practices (cGTP), and compliance with 21 CFR 1271.
Medical Device	510(k) Clearance	Generally requires "substantial equivalence" to a predicate device (510(k)). Clinical trials may or may not be required. Requires FDA current Good Manufacturing Practice (cGMP).
	Premarket Approval (PMA) Initial application is Investigational Device Exemption (IDE).	Extensive FDA premarket approval process, including comprehensive clinical trials. Conducted under Investigational Device Exemption (IDE). Requires FDA current Good Manufacturing Practice (cGMP). Safety and efficacy testing.
Biologic	Biologics License Application (BLA) Initial application is Investigational New Drug (IND).	Extensive FDA premarket approval process, including comprehensive preclinical and clinical trials. Requires compliance to FDA current Good Manufacturing Practice (cGMP). Safety and efficacy testing. Identity, purity, and potency requirements.
Drug	New Drug Application (NDA) Initial application is Investigational New Drug (IND).	Extensive FDA premarket approval process, including comprehensive clinical trials. Requires FDA Current Good Manufacturing Practice (cGMP). Safety and efficacy testing. Identity, purity, and potency requirements.

The regulatory complexity surrounding how products are classified, what degree of research is necessary behind each group and the level of studies involved is beyond the scope of this Primer, but these are important considerations in understanding whether a particular study is governed by which section of the regulatory environment.

8.1.3 RESEARCH DEFINED

What constitutes research? In the United States, whether or not something constitutes research has been well defined by the OHRP, and has been condensed into several spreadsheets available on that site (see http://www.hhs.gov/ohrp/policy/checklists/decisioncharts.html).[249] An example of the first spreadsheet is shown in Figure 44.

Additional direction at this site will permit the user to work through various potential exclusions or exemptions to the process, but generally, ***virtually all prospective clinical trials involving human subjects are defined as clinical research.***

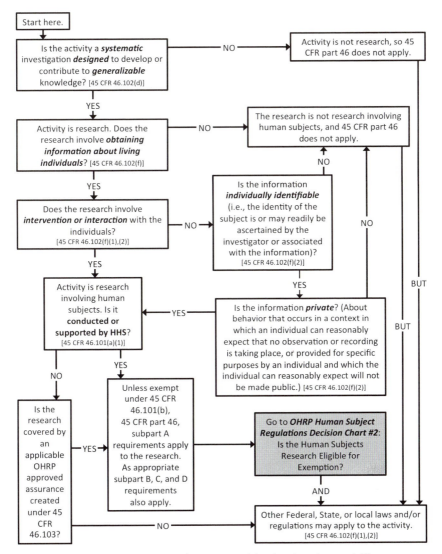

Figure 44. Example of a flowchart to determine if an activity is defined as clinical research.[249]

8.2 GOOD CLINICAL PRACTICES

The complete description of what constitutes appropriate clinical practices during research is beyond the scope of this chapter, but a number of key documents are typically compiled as part of a clinical research project. Most of these are addressed in the **ICH E6** guidance document and are standard components of clinical trials.

Systematic research involves the completion of various documents and processes. Key documents that are integral to the process include the following:

8.2.1 CLINICAL TRIAL PROTOCOL

The clinical trial protocol outlines the exact method by which the clinical trial will be conducted. Each clinical trial has an identified Principal Investigator and may also have Co-Investigators or Associate Investigators. Typical components of this document include the following components:

- Introduction
- Outline of the issue and experimental device or material
- Population addressed
- Inclusion/Exclusion criteria
- Outcome measures (primary measures, secondary measures)
- Statistical analysis including power analysis, sample size determination, etc.
- Handling of adverse events including reporting
- Timeline for the study and milestones
- Emergency contact information
- Assurance of study compliance by the Principal Investigator

Clinical research protocols for new biological products, drugs, or devices or for new uses of existing approved products must be filed as an Investigational New Drug (IND) or Investigational Device Exception (IDE) application through the appropriate FDA Center. These initial studies may be a Phase I safety study (with or without efficacy outcomes) or may be Phase I/II safety and efficacy studies, depending on the scope of work and intended outcomes. If warranted, the study of a product may be continued into follow-on Phases and larger studies with more patients and defined outcomes necessary to obtain product licensure. Licensure of a product so that it can be sold is done through an FDA process of scientific and regulatory review to evaluate the product's safety and effectiveness. The type of licensure path depends on the type of product. For Class III medical devices, a Premarket Approval (PMA) is sent through CDRH. Biological products are submitted to CBER or CDRH as a Biologics License Application (BLA). Drugs are submitted to CDER as a New Drug Application (NDA). Combination products will be assigned to one of the

FDA Centers to lead the review and representative(s) from other relevant Center(s) will be part of the review process. Before the trial can begin, specific information needs to be provided to the FDA, and the research study is posted on the NIH site, ClinicalTrials. gov.[250]

8.2.2 INFORMED CONSENT DOCUMENT

GCP requires that Investigators receive adequate training on performing the study, including obtaining Informed Consent, and that patients receive adequate information about the study, what is expected, and the risks of participating. A complete description of what is required is also available online at the OHRP website.[251] These sections and activities are expanded in special circumstances, such as emergency procedures, and studies with children, captive (e.g. prisoner) populations, mentally incompetent individuals, etc.

As dictated by the *Informed Consent Checklist – Basic and Additional Elements* (§46.116 of 45 CFR 46), formal informed consent documents typically have 12 or more sections, including the following general areas:[252]

- A statement that the study involves research
- An explanation of the purposes of the research
- The expected duration of the subject's participation
- A description of the procedures to be followed
- Identification of any procedures which are experimental
- A description of any reasonably foreseeable risks or discomforts to the subject
- A description of any benefits to the subject or to others who may reasonably be expected to benefit from the research
- A disclosure of appropriate alternative procedures or courses of treatment, if any, that might be advantageous to the subject
- A statement describing the extent, if any, to which confidentiality of records identifying the subject will be maintained
- For research involving more than minimal risk, an explanation as to whether any compensation, and an explanation as to whether any medical treatments are available, if injury occurs and, if so, what they consist of, or where further information may be obtained
- Research, Rights or Injury: An explanation of whom to contact for answers to pertinent questions about the research and research subjects' rights, and whom to contact in the event of a research-related injury to the subject
- A statement that participation is voluntary, refusal to participate will involve no penalty or loss of benefits to which the subject is otherwise entitled, and the

subject may discontinue participation at any time without penalty or loss of benefits, to which the subject is otherwise entitled

- A clearly indicated statement on disposition of any biological materials provided by the subject for the study. That is, must they be disposed of or can they be used for additional studies; and, if so, defining the conditions for use and storage.

8.2.3 INVESTIGATOR BROCHURE

Clinicians participating in a clinical trial are provided with detailed information about the material being tested, scientific basis for the study, and sufficient information to be able to run and monitor the study as a trained observer.

8.2.4 IRB EVALUATION AND APPROVAL

As required by law, an Institutional Review Board (IRB), which is an Independent Ethics Committee comprised of trained clinical and scientific investigators as well as community representative(s), reviews the protocol, informed consent, and related documents for all prospective clinical trials, and for all retrospective clinical trials where patient identification is possible. Regulation of IRB activity is a Federal responsibility and failure to comply with IRB processes is a Federal crime. IRB approval must be obtained before a trial can begin.

Interestingly, IRBs are set up mainly to confirm that a clinical trial is ethical and that the process will not harm patients. Whether or not the clinical trial is constructed properly or not is commented upon, but may not be a major focus of the review. For this reason, many institutions also require a concurrent review by an institutional "Office of Clinical Research" and a regular meeting of supervising clinicians during the process.

8.2.5 BUDGET DOCUMENTS

Typically, budget documents must be sufficiently well developed to avoid either monetary shortfall or accusations of improperly directing funds to researchers. The format of standard research financial pro forma documents create itemized lists of tasks and assigned expenses, each arrayed with a fair market value assignation. Use of generally accepted accounting principles in such documents also permits the correct assignment of capital expenditures, variable and fixed costs, etc.

Importantly, any payments to study subjects must be properly implemented and documented, and must stay in compliance with the informed consent and approved study documents.

8.2.6 OTHER DOCUMENTS AND LEGAL AGREEMENTS

Typically these may include a:

- Case Report Forms (CRF) forms and study forms used for the standardized collection of information such as patient demographics, outcome measures, etc.
- Primary source information documents.
- Nondisclosure agreement (NDA) between the researcher and the sponsoring organization to not reveal results or trade secrets.
- Study agreements with Investigators and/or Institutions to specifically define roles and responsibilities, funding, timelines, and deliverables.
- Intellectual property assignment.
- Technology transfer agreements.
- Materials storage and inventory management.
- Training records of Investigators and study staff.

8.3 PROJECT MANAGEMENT

8.3.1 PROJECT MANAGEMENT PROCESS

Proper execution of a clinical trial involves a number of steps. These may include:

- Detailed roles, responsibilities, timelines, and deliverables defined.
- Initial interactions with FDA as "pre-IND" or "pre-IDE" meetings for planning
- Planned, formal IND or IDE meetings with FDA (in person or via teleconference).
- Written IND or IDE and all support documents, including pre-clinical studies.
- Investigator site selection.
- Investigator training and Investigator brochure.
- IRB approval.
- Initial site and quality review visit.
- Periodic site monitoring visits.
- Formal site close out visits.
- Final site summary documents and IRB notification.
- Preparation and evaluation of primary source information.
- Generation of study reports.
- Final IRB filing and updates.
- Adverse event tracking and reporting.

8.3.2 PROJECT MANAGEMENT

Clinical trials, even small ones, involve multiple steps, regulatory requirements and individuals working across multiple areas of a company, research institution, or university environment. The identification of a single point of control (Project Manager) and responsibility for each task (Task Managers) facilitates the optimal management of the process. This is also facilitated using flow diagrams of processes with indicated timelines and responsibilities, and the use of Gantt charts to help assure that a project stays on track.

8.4 OUTCOMES ANALYSIS AND REPORTING

8.4.1 PRIMARY OUTCOME MEASURES

Outcomes reporting for clinical trials focus on a specific outcome measure, called the primary outcome measure, which addresses the principal question of the trial. This can take the form of answering the question "Is treatment X better than placebo?" (a *superiority trial*) or "Is treatment X the same as treatment Y?" (a *noninferiority trial*). Outcomes data are designed to be quantitative and are typically reported with assigned statistical significance using standard statistical terms such as p-value. Lack of statistical significance should also be reported.

8.4.2 SECONDARY OUTCOME MEASURES

Other outcomes are also reported, and can include both rigidly defined quantitative data with statistical outcomes, as well as observations and more intangible outcomes, although quantitative results are preferred.

8.4.3 PUBLICATION REQUIREMENTS

Increasingly, the submission of clinical research to legitimate medical journals has become more focused on the proper performance of research protocols. Virtually all articles submitted to major journals now require an IRB approval number for a clinical trial, or a formal IRB waiver of the need for an IRB approval, as well as registration of the study at ClinicalTrials.gov. Journals are also moving away from lower quality evidence and exhibiting preference for Level I and Level II clinical studies.

Medical journal articles are also moving to improved standards for reporting clinical results. The CONSORT criteria for example are followed by major medical journals and account for in the inclusion of selection flowcharts in clinical trial reporting for example.[253,254]

104

8.5 STATISTICAL ISSUES

Clinical trials are set up statistically to reduce the possibility of forming either a false positive (something works when it really doesn't) or false negative (something doesn't work when it really does) conclusion about the effectiveness of a treatment. The statistical analysis that accompanies clinical trials can be quite complex, but several key concepts are important for the proper study design and execution of a clinical trial.

8.5.1 BIAS

Bias is the tendency for observations or measurements to be influenced by factors outside of the experiment. Researchers try to remove sources of bias whenever possible. Observer bias might occur when a researcher wants something to work very badly, to validate an invention or theory, or clinical result. Patients can often bias results if they are aware of what treatment is used, experiencing a higher rate of side effects for example. Other biases can be statistical or unrelated to the observer, such as coming to a different conclusion because the subjects were younger and healthier than what might be expected, or if they were consistently of a lower socioeconomic status. Bias is removed by blinding the patient and researcher/observer when possible, by creating a randomized clinical trial, and by administering the study over many geographically dispersed sites and with different investigators.

8.5.2 P-VALUE

A common statistic that is used to determine whether there is a difference between a treatment group and a control group is the p-value. This statistical term is a calculated number that describes the possibility that the outcomes may have occurred based on chance alone. The number typically used to validate clinical research are values less than or equal to 0.05. Differences can be seen between any two populations where a number of tests are taken, but to have value, a conclusion must be statistically significant.

8.5.3 POWER ANALYSIS

Because of this issue, and before undertaking a clinical study, researchers must understand what differences they expect to find at least generally between the treatment under consideration and the control or comparison group. A power analysis is done using estimates of the effect size of the treatment in the population to determine the number of subjects necessary to be able to demonstrate a statistically significant result. Typically, the smaller the effect size, the larger the population is necessary to prove statistical significance. If a study is "underpowered" results will be achieved but may not be "statistically significant" due to an insufficient population size. Observed differences cannot be stated as significant. Statistical inference is difficult though when the effect size is small and there is not much difference between the test material or drug and the effects of the Standard of Care. Statistical power is dependent on both the number of subjects enrolled and the degree to which patients treated with a certain therapy show a difference in the primary outcome measure used.

In the end, statistical analysis will come to a conclusion about the research that shows whether an effect is present or not. It may also guide the decision on whether or not multiple or additional trials be conducted to confirm the clinical impression of an effect.

8.6 EVALUATION OF RESEARCH: EVALUATING THE QUALITY OF REPORTED CLINICAL TRIAL OUTCOMES

The literature is filled with articles and research where proper principles of study construction were not followed or the results not correctly interpreted, either inadvertently or intentionally. What might one look for when examining published studies to determine the most appropriate level of truth?

8.6.1 LEVELS OF EVIDENCE

As a way of establishing the relationship between a therapy and the likelihood that it is effective and safe, clinicians have developed the term *evidence based medicine* to define this process, and have created a hierarchy of describing the validity and reliability of the studies involved.

Since clinical experiments can be conducted in an almost unlimited number of ways, clinical scientists have created a hierarchy to define the relative strength of various approaches. Called "Levels of Evidence," this approach ranks clinical trials into several categories. Expressed as an ascending level of increasing reliability, clinical studies are sorted into increasingly strong validation tiers confirming their results. These include the following levels generally, although other methods and modifications have been proposed and are used in various environments.[255,256]

Table X. Levels of evidence to classify the strength and reliability of clinical studies.

LEVEL OF EVIDENCE	DEFINITION/DESCRIPTION
Level I	High quality, formal randomized controlled clinical trials (RCTs) or reviews of RCTs.
Level II	High quality systematic case controlled trials where comparisons with a matched or balanced group are made but not randomized.
Level III	Observational studies such as case studies, surveys and questionnaires.
Level IV	Expert opinion, independent user evaluations and reviews.

Key terms needed to understand this approach include the following;

- ***Randomized*** = patients are placed into one of two or more groups by random assignment, for example to receive either an active drug or a placebo.
- ***Controlled*** = assignment of subjects is controlled by a process that fairly assigns potential candidates and prevents self-selection or similar biases from affecting the randomization process.
- ***Blinded*** = prevention of a tested individual from knowing what treatment is given (***single blind***) or the individual and the treating clinician from knowing what treatment was applied (***double blind***).

Clinical trials are well known to suffer sometimes very subtle biases based on the conditions of patient selection, physician preferences and opinions, etc. The placebo effect is very strong, causing patients to improve with treatments they believe will be beneficial. Controlling the assignment of patients into various treatment groups and blinding them to which therapy is used prevents inadvertent biases from influencing the results that might occur in case reports or the observations of individual observers.

A student of the literature will note that various groups may further subdivide these categories in different ways, but the concept of progressive reliability of the evidence is the essential concept.[255,256]

8.6.2 CONFLICT OF INTEREST

The current medical environment may find clinicians in a position that their positive support of a study result or a particular product results in substantial personal benefit to themselves. This can hardly be avoided with prominent researchers, of course, but the degree to which a significant conflict of interest can occur should always be evaluated. Clinicians who are "company spokespersons" for many years may be suspect, for example, but can be acceptable. Over the past twenty to thirty years, the federal government has implemented a number of very stringent laws designed to suppress self-referral, kickbacks, and inappropriate conflict of interest by investigators. Recent Office of the Inspector General (OIG) regulations are further restricting even individuals at an arm's length from actual researchers such as paid corporate medical directors who are also clinically in practice.

Generally, results of medical research are most robust if they have been conducted by non-conflicted researchers in an approach that creates Level I results in a multicenter, repeatable manner using Good Clinical Practices and has been formally approved by an Institutional Review Board. Expectation for and use of the CONSORT reporting format is another method to minimize the likelihood of misleading results. Conversely, research that is improperly constructed, without IRB approval and/or with minimal regard to Good Clinical Practices, should be considered highly suspect and potentially unreliable.

CHAPTER 9

MIMEDX SCIENTIFIC PUBLICATIONS

MiMedx is committed to, and is actively involved in, state of the art scientific research directed towards a complete understanding of the mechanisms of action underlying the clinical effectiveness of its PURION Processed dehydrated human amnion chorion membrane allografts (dHACM). Analytical biochemical methods are used to characterize graft composition, especially related to inherent growth factors, cytokines, and chemokines. Each of the phases of physiological healing – inflammation, proliferation and remodeling – requires the coordinated participation of a suite of specific cell types, including cells of the immune system, fibroblasts, endothelial cells, and hematopoietic and mesenchymal stem cells. Therefore, *in vitro* cell culture is often used as a targeted model system to investigate and delineate the effects of dHACM on the metabolic activities of human cells critically involved in wound healing and tissue regeneration. Also ischemic murine models are employed to evaluate the effect of dHACM *in vivo* on cellular activities during healing.

Using the techniques described previously, **seven peer-reviewed articles have been published since 2012** examining the *in vitro* and *in vivo* effects of PURION Processed dHACM on cellular responses.[73-79] In addition, **over fifteen additional peer-reviewed articles have been published since 2012** reporting the clinical efficacy of PURION Processed dHACM in a variety of wounds.[47,80-94] By comparison, competitive products average less than one peer-reviewed scientific or clinical publication each, and most have none. The following provides a brief summary of the salient conclusions and interpretations from these studies with a focus on critical cell-mediated mechanisms inherent to the process of healing. PURION Processed dHACM was used in these studies; therefore, the following results apply only to PURION Processed dHACM allografts, as correlation to allografts processed using alternative techniques has not been demonstrated.

9.1 CYTOKINE CONTENT IN MIMEDX dHACM GRAFTS

Over 226 growth factors, cytokines, chemokines, and regulatory proteins were identified in MiMedx PURION Processed dHACM tissues to date.[73-75,237] These molecules, which include growth factors, immunomodulatory cytokines and chemokines, and TIMPs, possess important regulatory roles in modulating various stages of tissue healing and regeneration. The dHACM allografts act by delivering these molecules into the hydrated wound environment. It was demonstrated that a fraction of these molecules are freely soluble and elute out of the tissue in hydrated environments, while the remaining fraction remains bound within the extracellular matrix until released by tissue degradation.[74]

Inflammation is critical during the early stages of wound repair; therefore, a balance of immunoregulatory proteins may be crucial signals to support healing of wounds. The dHACM contains inflammatory cell chemokines and cytokines that regulate the activity of cells derived from the immune system. Chemokines recruit immune cells to the site of a wound, and cytokines regulate activity of these immune cells. The dHACM contains chemokines and cytokines that directly affect T-cells, B lymphocytes, monocytes and macrophages, neutrophils, eosinophils, and natural killer cells. Together this balance of inflammatory regulators modulates the inflammation response within healing wounds, and together with additional wound healing cytokines also retained in PURION Processed dHACM provides an ideal balance of cues to promote healing.[74]

The dHACM contains both amnion and chorion layers of the amniotic membrane, and it was determined that amnion and chorion tissues contained similar amounts of growth factors when normalized per dry weight; however, when calculated per surface area of tissue applied to a wound, chorion contained on average three to four times more of each factor than the amnion, due to the greater thickness of the chorion membrane.[76] Therefore, an allograft containing both amnion and chorion would contain four to five times more cytokines than a single layer amnion allograft alone. Additionally, MiMedx PURION processed single layer amnion grafts contained significantly more cytokines than other single layer products that have been analyzed.[76] These results suggest that PURION Processed dHACM contains substantially more cytokines than these other single layer amnion products, and the PURION Process retains greater cytokine content than the other commercial tissue processing methods studied, even when only comparing single layer amnion products.[104] Therefore, not all amniotic membrane allografts are created equally, and **the PURION Process provides a distinct advantage over the other amniotic membrane allografts processed using alternative techniques, by retaining and preserving the high concentration of cytokines found in the amniotic**

membrane. MiMedx PURION Processed dHACM has also been demonstrated through various published clinical studies to be an effective treatment to promote wound healing, perhaps due to high concentrations and a vast array of various growth factors delivered to the wound.[47,80-94]

9.2 MIMEDX dHACM PROMOTES CELL PROLIFERATION

When soluble extracts of MiMedx dHACM tissue, which contain the various growth factors and cytokines discussed above, were applied to cells *in vitro*, PURION Processed dHACM was shown to stimulate proliferation in a variety of cells relevant to healing and repair. These cells included human dermal fibroblasts, microvascular endothelial cells, mesenchymal stem cells, adipose derived stem cells, and hematopoietic stem cells.[73,75,78,104] These results showed that dHACM directly causes cells to proliferate *in vitro* by releasing growth factors that activate the proliferative response. Proliferation of these cells amplifies the respective population of these cells in the wounds, thus increasing their regenerative potential. HDF proliferation is a critical part of wound closure and tissue replacement, HMVE proliferation is directly correlated to neovascularization within the healing tissue, and stem cell proliferation enhances the reparative signaling and regenerative capabilities of these cells.

9.3 MIMEDX dHACM ACTS AS A "STEM CELL MAGNET" TO PROMOTE CELL RECRUITMENT

In addition to promoting cell proliferation, PURION Processed dHACM was shown to recruit migration of adult stem cells, including mesenchymal stem cells, adipose derived stem cells, and hematopoietic stem cells *in vitro* and *in vivo*. Using *in vitro* assays, MSCs migrated across porous membranes toward pieces of dHACM tissue,[73] and MSCs and ADSCs migrated to accelerate closure of cell-free zones in the presence of soluble dHACM extracts, comparable to closure of acellular wounds.[78] To confirm these observations *in vivo*, two murine ischemic skin wound models of stem cell migration were also used. Following subcutaneous implantation, greater numbers of bone marrow MSCs and HSCs were measured at the site of dHACM implantation in wild type mice.[73,77] Additionally, using a GFP parabiosis model, GFP+ bone marrow stem cells were identified at sites of neovascularization within the implanted dHACM grafts, indicating that stem cells were recruited from the bone marrow stem cell niche toward the dHACM grafts through the blood circulation.[77] When compared to control graft tissue composed of acellular fetal dermal matrix (ADM, PriMatrix, TEI Biosciences), PURION Processed dHACM stimulated recruit greater levels of stem cell recruitment than the ADM tissue.

Additionally, dHACM implantation upregulated cellular expression of stromal derived factor 1α (SDF-1α), a known stem cell recruiting factor, which may attract additional cells to the site and further promote repair.[77] Together, these data indicate that dHACM recruits circulatory stem and progenitor cells toward sites of implantation within healing wounds, providing a partial mechanism for the clinical efficacy of human amniotic membrane in the treatment of wounds.

Stem and progenitor cells play vital roles in normal tissue maintenance, as well as wound repair and tissue regeneration. Mesenchymal stem cells are pivotal cells that are normally recruited to sites of injury, where they mount a multifaceted cascade regulating inflammatory mechanisms, angiogenesis, and tissue regeneration. These results indicate that dHACM may stimulate healing by recruiting mesenchymal stem cells to revitalize a wound. PURION Processed dHACM delivers soluble stem cell recruiting factors that cause human MSCs and HSCs to migrate towards the graft, acting as a ***stem cell magnet*** to amplify stem cell populations within healing wounds, as depicted in Figure 45. This presents a novel technique to repopulate a wound with regenerative stem cells by recruiting them from the patient's own reservoir of active stem cells. Subsequently, the stem cells may engraft in the wound and modulate the wound environment to promote progression down the natural healing pathway. Stem cell recruitment of the patient's own stem cells into the wound is a contrasting approach to live cell therapies, which intend to deliver live allogeneic cells into the harsh wound environment. It has been widely

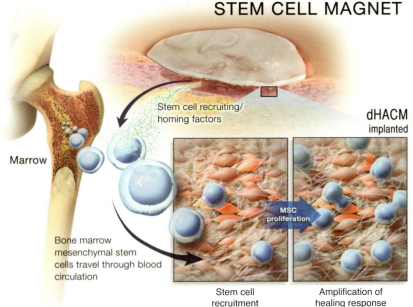

Figure 45. dHACM acts as a stem cell magnet to recruit stem cells to the injured tissue.[73,77]

shown that a major limitation of live cell therapies is that very few of the delivered cells engraft, remain viable, and persist in a wound within several days,[41-43] suggesting that stem cell recruitment of endogenous cells may be a promising approach to modulate stem cell activity and promote healing and repair. **Therefore, PURION Processed dHACM acts as stem cell magnet to recruit stem cells and amplify stem cell populations within healing wounds, and the ability to recruit stem cells has not been demonstrated in any other amniotic membrane allografts.**

9.4 MIMEDX dHACM ALTERS SECRETION OF IMMUNOMODULATORY, ANGIOGENIC, AND TISSUE PROMOTING CYTOKINES

While repopulating wounded tissues through cell proliferation and migration, PURION Processed dHACM has also been shown to stimulate secretion of cytokines by cells, including secretion of immunomodulatory, angiogenic, and tissue growth promoting cytokines by fibroblasts, vascular endothelial cells, and stem cells. When treated with dHACM extracts, human dermal fibroblasts upregulated biosynthesis of bFGF, GCSF, and PlGF *in vitro*, three growth factors involved in healing.[74] Similarly, dHACM treatment induced production of over 30 angiogenic factors by human microvascular endothelial cells *in vitro*, including granulocyte macrophage colony-stimulating factor (GM-CSF), angiogenin, transforming growth factor β3 (TGF-β3), and HB-EGF.[75]

The role of stem cells in healing has also focused on the paracrine signaling properties of these cells, including their influence on the inflammatory status of injured tissues.[257] ADSCs, BM-MSCs, and HSCs were shown to modulate secretion of a number of cytokines involved in immunoregulation and mitogenesis in response to dHACM extracts. Of these molecules, they can generally be classified into three unique functions: 1) chemokines and proteins related to leukocyte migration, 2) immunomodulatory cytokines, and 3) mitogenic growth factors and proteins related to tissue growth.[78]

Upregulated chemokines, including I-309, IL-8, IL-16, MCP-1, MIP-1α, and MIP-1β, are known to direct chemotaxis of immune cells that are critical in healing, including monocytes and macrophages, neutrophils, T lymphocytes, dendritic cells, and eosinophils.[7] Similarly ICAM-1, which was upregulated in all three stem cell types, is an adhesion molecule that facilitates leukocyte endothelial transmigration,[258] suggesting a potential role of ICAM-1 in the extravasation of circulating stem cells from the blood vessels toward the dHACM treated site. In wound settings, these chemokines are commonly expressed early following establishment of hemostasis, often peaking at day 1 with expression sustained through the first week of healing, and have also been shown to promote angiogenesis.[7] Immunomodulatory cytokines, including GDF-15, IL-

1Ra, and IL-6, were also upregulated in MSCs, ADSCs, and HSCs. These cytokines are known to regulate various pro- and anti-inflammatory cues that are required for healing, including regulation of apoptosis, T cell activation, B cell differentiation, macrophage differentiation, hematopoiesis, and additional downstream immunomodulatory cues.[181,259,260] Additionally, growth factors and growth factor regulatory molecules, including EGF, FGF-4, GH, IGFBP-1, IGFBP-2, and SCF, were secreted in response to dHACM. These growth cytokines are known to stimulate cell proliferation, migration, differentiation, cell survival, and protein synthesis, and have been shown to enhance healing of wounds.[223,224,261,262] Finally, TIMP-1, which was also upregulated, is an inhibitor of MMPs and is actively involved in tissue remodeling processes.[263]

These results indicate that in addition to the growth factors and cytokines released from dHACM tissue into the wound, dHACM continues to amplify these paracrine signals by inducing resident cells to produce additional regenerative growth factors, thus enhancing dHACM's regenerative effect. Together this balance of regulatory signals modulates the healing response to provide an ideal balance of cues to promote healing.

9.5 MIMEDX dHACM PROMOTES ANGIOGENESIS

Angiogenesis, or the creation of new blood vessels, is paramount during the late inflammatory and proliferative phases of wound healing since chronic wounds are commonly associated with poor circulation and vascularization. The following angiogenic cytokines were identified to be intrinsically present in PURION Processed dHACM: angiogenin, angiopoietin-2 (ANG-2), epidermal growth factor (EGF), basic fibroblast growth factor (bFGF), heparin binding epidermal growth factor (HB-EGF), hepatocyte growth factor (HGF), platelet derived growth factor BB (PDGF-BB), placental growth factor (PlGF), and vascular endothelial growth factor (VEGF). The dHACM had a direct effect on stimulating human dermal microvascular endothelial cells. dHACM caused HMVE cells to proliferate, recruited migration of endothelial cells, and induced production of over 30 angiogenic factors by these cells *in vitro*, including granulocyte macrophage colony-stimulating factor (GM-CSF), angiogenin, transforming growth factor β3 (TGF-β3), and HB-EGF.[75]

In an *in vivo* murine ischemic wound model, a steady increase in microvessels was observed in dHACM implants over a 4 week period to levels equivalent to healthy and healed skin, indicative of a dynamic intra-dHACM implant neovascular process.[75] Recruited bone marrow stem cells were also localized to sites of neovascularization within the implanted graft where they expressed angiogenic stromal derived factor 1α (SDF-1α).[77] Taken together, these results demonstrate that **MiMedx PURION Processed dHACM grafts: 1) contain angiogenic growth factors retaining biological activity; 2)** promote amplification of angiogenic cues by inducing endothelial cell proliferation and migration and by upregulating production of endogenous angiogenic growth factors by endothelial cells; and 3) support the formation of blood vessels *in vivo*, as shown in Figure 46.

These results indicate that MiMedx dHACM stimulates angiogenesis when applied to a wound through the presence of angiogenic factors coupled with dHACM's effect on the production of angiogenic factors by endothelial cells. The effect of dHACM is amplified by increasing the number of endothelial cells in the wound via migration and proliferation and by inducing cells to produce additional angiogenic factors to produce a potent local angiogenic environment.

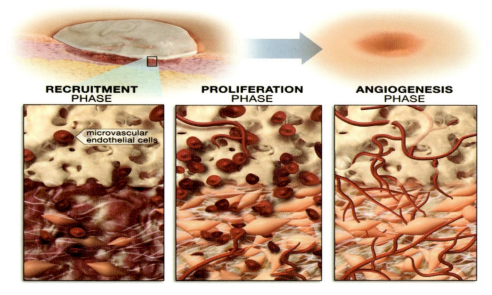

Figure 46. dHACM promotes angiogenesis in injured tissue.[75,77]

9.6 MIMEDX dHACM DEMONSTRATES BIOLOGICAL ACTIVITY IN STEM CELLS FROM DIABETIC PATIENTS

In diabetes, hyperglycemia caused by decreased insulin availability or increased resistance to insulin can negatively affect the cellular response to tissue injury, resulting in chronic wounds that are stalled in a state of chronic inflammation and unable to progress toward healing. This may be due in part to the impaired responsiveness of reparative stem cells at the wound. The diabetes-induced state of hyperglycemia has been linked to having a deleterious effect on wound healing associated with changes in ADSC cellular morphology, decreased proliferation and migration and abnormal cellular differentiation.[264,265] The altered pattern of growth factor and cytokine levels in diabetes may also contribute to the cellular complications seen in chronic wound tissues.[266] Reduced bioavailability of cytokines and growth factors such as vascular endothelial growth factor (VEGF), basic fibroblast growth factor (bFGF), transforming growth factor alpha (TGF-α) and platelet derived growth factor (PDGF) have been implicated in the pathogenesis of chronic wounds,[267] and abnormal expression of growth factors has been reported in studies of diabetic foot ulcer tissues.[268]

Despite these impaired cellular responses in diabetic tissues, the eluted soluble growth factors and cytokines from dHACM were capable of stimulating ADSCs from Type I and Type II diabetic donors to proliferate, migrate, and modulate gene expression and secretion of immunomodulatory cytokines *in vitro.*[79] Type I and Type II diabetic ADSCs increased secretion of the immunomodulatory factors IL-6, IL-8, MCP-1, MIP-1b and RANTES and upregulated gene expression of IL-1α, IL-1β, and IL-1Ra, which are responsible for the inflammatory regulation functionality of ADSCs in wound healing.[269] These immunomodulatory cytokines are essential for normal progression through wound healing. Thus, initial upregulation of certain pro-inflammatory factors through treatment with dHACM may be necessary for resetting the cascade of normal healing in a chronic wound. Ultimately, regulation of, as opposed to elimination of, immunomodulatory cytokines by ADSCs is crucial for re-establishing or resetting an acute wound healing trajectory.

The results presented here demonstrate that while ADSCs from diabetic donors can have decreased capacities for proliferation and migration as well as altered cytokine secretion profiles compared to normal ADSCs, stem cells derived from diabetic patients were capable of responding to treatment with MiMedx PURION Processed dHACM. Type I and Type II diabetic ADSCs increased proliferation in response to dHACM, increased cellular migration in response to soluble factors eluted from dHACM tissue, and altered their immunomodulatory cytokine secretion and gene expression to produce a number of factors important to healing of chronic wounds, representing a first step in determining how stem cells in diabetic patients may respond to dHACM treatment to promote healing of chronic wounds.

9.7 SCIENTIFIC DATA ARE SUPPORTED BY MIMEDX dHACM'S PROVEN CLINICAL EFFICACY

Scientific experiments continue to generate new information in order to elucidate potential cellular and molecular mechanisms through which dHACM grafts promote healing. MiMedx has published several papers to date in peer reviewed journals that establish that MiMedx PURION Processed amniotic tissues (e.g., EpiFix and AmnioFix) retain over 50 regulatory proteins, including cytokines, chemokines and growth factors that are naturally present in fresh amniotic membrane.[73-75] Those studies demonstrate that PURION Processed amniotic tissues retain biologically active signals that directly cause responsive cells to proliferate, upregulate biosynthesis of important growth factors and immunomodulatory regulators, recruit mesenchymal stem cell migration towards the allograft, and enhance angiogenesis within healing wounds *in vitro* and *in vivo*.[73-75,77-79]

These cellular responses were demonstrated using MiMedx PURION Processed dHACM; however, all amniotic membrane allografts are not equal, and similar biological responses have not been demonstrated in any other tissue allografts. In contrast, competitive tissue allograft products studied have been shown to contain only a fraction of the soluble factors that are retained in dHACM through the PURION Process.[76] These wound care products also have not demonstrated the wealth of scientific data or clinical healing results established by MiMedx. Due to the decreased growth factor and cytokine content in these grafts, the competitive allograft tissues studied would not be expected to possess the same ability to modulate cell responses and stimulate healing as MiMedx's PURION Processed tissues.

Figures 47 and 48 demonstrate the increased rate of healing of MiMedx PURION Processed dHACM over Standard of Care treatment, as well as Organogenesis Apligraf bioengineered skin substitute.[47,80] In a prospective, randomized clinical trial, Zelen et al. demonstrated a significant increase in the healing rate of diabetic foot ulcers with biweekly application of MiMedx PURION Processed dHACM, compared to those treated with a standard therapeutic regimen (moist wound therapy), with 77% and 92% of dHACM wounds healed at week 4 and 6, respectively, compared to only 0% and 8% of controls (Figure 47).[80] Additionally, wounds that healed after dHACM treatment did not recur with long-term follow-up,[81] and in a crossover study of patients that failed to heal with standard care treatment, 55% demonstrated complete healing by 4 weeks, 64% by 6 weeks, and 91% by 12 weeks with biweekly application of PURION Processed dHACM.[83] When compared to Organogenesis Apligraf bioengineered skin substitute, 85% and 95% of DFUs treated MiMedx PURION Processed dHACM achieved complete wound closure within 4 and 6 weeks, respectively, which was significantly higher than for patients receiving Apligraf (35% and 45%, respectively) or standard care treatment with collagen-alginate dressing (30% and 35%, respectively).[47]

These *in vitro* and *in vivo* scientific results strongly suggest that PURION Processed dHACM is intimately involved with modulation of the cellular environments in wounds to elicit an improved healing response, and the reparative attributes of dHACM allografts are further supported by the numerous peer reviewed published clinical trials on their use on diabetic foot ulcers and venous leg ulcers, as well as initial investigations in plantar fasciitis, tympanoplasty (surgical eardrum repair), transforaminal lumbar interbody fusion of the spine, and osteoarthritis.[47,80-94] These clinical trials clearly demonstrate a more rapid rate of healing in dHACM treated wounds, compared to Standard of Care, indicating that PURION Processed dHACM modulates inflammation and promotes improved tissue growth.[80,81,83,84,93]

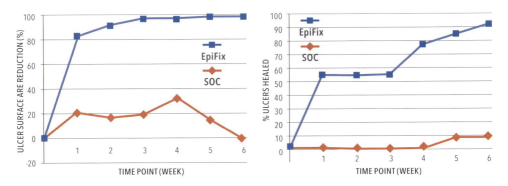

Figure 47. EpiFix dHACM promotes wound healing of diabetic ulcers. Percent reduction in diabetic foot ulcer surface area (left panel) and percent of ulcers healed (right panel) following dHACM treatment, compared to Standard of Care treatment of moist wound therapy.[80]

Mean % Wound Area Healed per Week

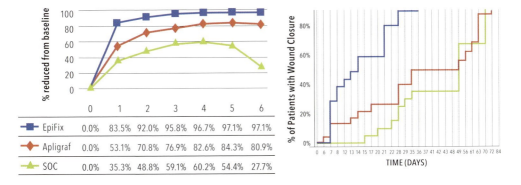

Figure 48. EpiFix dHACM outperforms Apligraf and Standard of Care in promoting wound healing of diabetic ulcers. Percent reduction in diabetic lower extremity ulcer surface area (left panel) and speed to healing (right panel) with dHACM treatment, compared to Organogenesis Apligraf bioengineered skin substitute and Standard of Care treatment with collagen-alginate dressing.[47]

In summary, the wealth of scientific knowledge compiled by MiMedx suggests that PURION Processed dHACM releases soluble signals into the wound environment that promote cell proliferation, migration, and endogenous cytokine secretion and ultimately stimulates stem cell activity, angiogenesis, and modulation of inflammation to support healing.

CHAPTER 10

MIMEDX CLINICAL STUDIES, RANDOMIZED CONTROLLED TRIALS, AND PUBLISHED LITERATURE

In an ongoing commitment to develop and establish the scientific basis of its product portfolio, MiMedx has undertaken a systematic approach to documenting the clinical value of EpiFix and AmnioFix, its dehydrated human amnion/chorion membrane (dHACM) products. This has resulted in an extensive collection of clinical case material, formal clinical studies, and formal scientific publications in the indexed, peer-reviewed medical literature.

The clinical application of amniotic membranes dates back over one hundred years. MiMedx has accumulated a large library of literature on the placenta, including textbooks and over 300 articles on the medical applications of amniotic membrane for various indications. This literature forms a compelling historical base for the clinical use of amniotic membrane that is further expanded upon by MiMedx product-specific scientific and clinical support.

Initial clinical distribution of the company's products began with the application of amniotic membrane in eye surgery in 2006. By 2015, over 70,000 allografts have been distributed for eye surgery. Used in anterior reconstructive surgery for conjunctival and corneal repairs, these allografts are now the Standard of Care in those cases, with a formal reimbursement pathway that is well established. Similarly, the membrane has also been distributed widely for use by dental specialists, with application in periodontal reconstruction and repair. In addition, increased adoption and wide usage by wound and surgical specialists has resulted in over 450,000 PURION Processed allografts distributed to date.

10.1 MEDICAL LITERATURE FOR MIMEDX PRODUCTS

A growing body of literature has evolved surrounding the various applications of MiMedx's products for various other medical conditions. A listing of these articles is attached in Appendix A. Note that the broad range of uses for the material includes not only wound therapies, but treatments in ophthalmology, orthopedics, otorhinolaryngology, dermatology, dentistry, and other areas.

In 2011, an overview of the clinical uses of amniotic membrane was published by Donald Fetterolf, MD, Chief Medical Officer of MiMedx and Robert Snyder, DPM, then the Chief Podiatry Officer of the Diversified Clinical Services wound clinic organization in the journal Wounds. This important summary represents an introduction to not only the medical uses of amniotic membrane but its application in healing wounds in particular.[88] In this article the long history of amniotic membrane use in various wounds and the growing knowledge of the underlying scientific principles that define its mechanism of action were thoroughly discussed.

With well over 300 patients with chronic wounds treated across multiple randomized controlled trials, and at a number of clinical research locations, the clinical effectiveness of MiMedx PURION Processed dHACM for enhanced wound and soft tissue healing has been firmly established. Publications in peer reviewed journals confirm that the well-known healing properties of natural multi-layer amniotic membrane persist in the MiMedx multilayer PURION Processed allografts.

MiMedx first described the clinical effectiveness of its PURION Processed EpiFix dHACM membrane in the treatment of wounds through a series of case reports or case series published in the clinical literature.

10.2 EARLY CLINICAL CASE SERIES

Soon after its introduction as a potential treatment for wounds, clinical reports and case series that documented the impressive clinical effectiveness of these allografts were collected by MiMedx. Highlights of these clinical reports include:

Published Case Series by Alap Shah, DPM (Published in Journal of the American Podiatric Medical Association, JAPMA, 2014)

An initial case series originally conducted by Dr. Alap Shah, DPM, was published in the Journal of the American Podiatric Medical Association (JAPMA). In this publication, Dr. Shah describes a successful initial experience with EpiFix dHACM in treating various lower extremity ulcers.[89]

Published Case Series by Emran Sheikh, MD, MBA (Published in International Wound Journal, 2013)

Dr. Emran Sheikh, MD, MBA published a series of plastic surgery cases that were originally referred for skin grafting, in which EpiFix dHACM was applied instead.[85] Using wound size as a method of measuring wound responsiveness to therapy, Dr. Sheikh developed the graphical presentation of rapid healing in otherwise chronic wounds illustrated below in Figure 49.

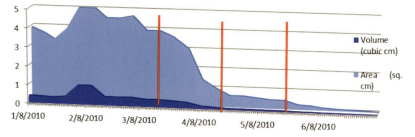

Figure 49. Healing rate in Case #2 patient in the article. MiMedx EpiFix dHACM was applied three times, on 3/17 (14wks), 4/22 (20wks), and 5/27 (25wks). (Red lines indicate applications of EpiFix). Rapid reductions in wound size with EpiFix application are noted.

Published Case Series by Jason Forbes, MD (Published in Journal of Wound Care, 2013)

A second case series was published by wound physician, Dr. Jason Forbes, MD. This series outlined the use of EpiFix in a variety of clinical wound settings in various locations.[86] The rapid healing kinetic curves for these patients led to the design of subsequent randomized clinical trials. Representative wound healing curves for the refractory ulcers that had been referred to the clinics are shown below in Figure 50.

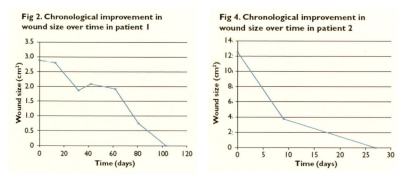

Figure 50. Representative wound healing curves for refractory ulcers in two patients over time following treatment with EpiFix.

Overall, well documented case series demonstrate healing properties of MiMedx PURION Processed dHACM material that were clearly superior to Standard of Care approaches.

10.3 RANDOMIZED CONTROLLED TRIALS

Zelen, C; Serena, T; Denoziere, G; Fetterolf, D. A prospective randomized comparative parallel study of amniotic membrane wound graft in the management of diabetic foot ulcers. (Published in International Wound Journal, 2013)

The first randomized controlled trial (RCT) examined the use of MiMedx EpiFix dHACM in patients with lower extremity diabetic ulcers, a particularly difficult wound type typically characterized by chronicity and long healing times.[80] The study was a single center, randomized, placebo controlled trial conducted by Dr. Charles Zelen at the Professional Education and Research Institute in Roanoke, VA. Patients with diabetic foot ulcers were treated with either Standard of Care (moist dressing changes) alone or Standard of Care and EpiFix applied every two weeks. The objective was to compare the reduction of wound size and proportion of wounds healed at 4 and 6 weeks. The secondary objectives were to measure the mean time to healing and the cost effectiveness of the two protocols of care.

The initial effect on wound reduction was so significant that the trial was terminated early at 25 patients. Results indicated a markedly different healing rate between the treatment and control groups, as outlined in the results published in the International Wound Journal.[80] It was initially felt by the investigator that further progression in the study by patients would be potentially unethical given this significant difference. Statistically the results were significant at small sample size due to the large healing effect of dHACM when compared to a moist saline Standard of Care control. Since this was larger than expected, the study achieved a high level of statistical significance with a much lower number of subjects, which were otherwise matched across study groups. The final results reported in the paper showed a high level of statistical significance:

"Patients were randomized to receive standard of care alone or standard of care with the addition of EpiFix. Wound size reduction and rates of complete healing after 4 and 6 weeks were evaluated. In the standard care group (n =12) and the EpiFix group (n =13) wounds reduced in size by a mean of 32.0% ± 47.3% versus 97.1% ± 7.0% (p <0.001) after 4 weeks, whereas at 6 weeks wounds were reduced by −1.8% +/-0.3% versus 98.4% ± 5.8% (p <0.001), standard care versus EpiFix, respectively. After 4 and 6 weeks of treatment the overall healing rate with application of EpiFix was shown to be 77% and 92%, respectively, whereas standard care healed 0% and 8% of the wounds (p<0.001), respectively. Patients treated with EpiFix achieved superior healing rates over standard treatment alone. These results show that using EpiFix in addition to standard care is efficacious for wound healing."

As an added measure and to confirm the remarkable initial results, the full series of patient photographs and wound measurements were reviewed by two independent nationally recognized wound surgeons, Thomas Serena, MD, current President of the American Professional Wound Care Association and Jason Hanft, DPM, a widely published wound specialist. Their review of the material confirmed the findings of

Dr. Zelen and resulted in early termination of the study. Results of the study noted a significant difference between Standard of Care and the treatment group, the large effect size creating a high level of statistical significance with these 25 patients (p<0.001).

Graphical representation of the wound healing kinetics is self-explanatory, and demonstrates a striking effect on wound size over time with biweekly application of dHACM (EpiFix), as shown in Figure 51:

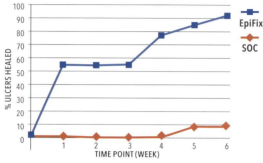

Figure 51. Comparison of wound surface area reduction from baseline for patients receiving the Standard of Care and for patients after the application of EpiFix.

Reviewers examining the study noted in particular that the normally chaotic wound size variation seen in many wound populations was absent in the EpiFix population, where dramatic wound size reductions were evident across the treatment group, as shown in Figure 52.

The chaotic nature of wound size over time has been identified in the past as a potential source of error in small trial size studies. For example, a randomly selected group of wounds receiving a particular therapy may identify a group that improves on its own as might be seen in a selected few of the Standard of Care patients in this study. However, noting the systematic and sustained response in EpiFix patients compared with the Standard of Care makes this visibly less likely as a possibility, and confirms the statistical conclusions and power/significance analysis.

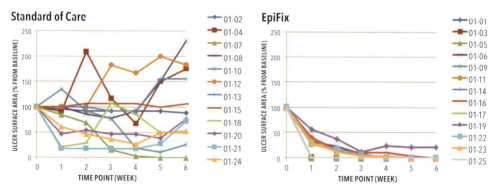

Figure 52. Comparison of wound surface area reduction from baseline for patients receiving the Standard of Care or EpiFix. Note that fluctuation in wound size typically seen in patients with these wounds treated with Standard of Care. When EpiFix is applied, a consistent reduction in size over time is noted.

It is also of interest that the Standard of Care patients, when crossed over to the EpiFix therapy, again move from the chaotic pattern of wound sizes over time to the same kinetic appearance of the treatment group. This is further confirmation that the effect size noted in these patients is robust across time and that the response to EpiFix treatment was relatively consistent compared to Standard of Care.

Zelen, C. An evaluation of dehydrated human amniotic membrane allografts in patients with DFUs. (Published in Journal of Wound Care, 2013)

As part of the above study, the anticipated nonresponse of the control group patients presented an opportunity for demonstrating the effectiveness of EpiFix dHACM in these patients when they were subsequently treated with this material after leaving the study, essentially creating an N of 1 style case series crossover component to the study. A similar notable healing response of these patients was also documented by the investigator; these results were published in a peer reviewed medical journal as well.[83] The 11 patients in the crossover study demonstrated the same rapid healing kinetics, with 88% of the patients eventually healing within 9 weeks as shown in Table XI and Figure 53.

Table XI. Table indicating original and crossover EpiFix treated patients.

GROUP	INITIAL NUMBER	HEAL 6 WEEKS	HEAL 9 WEEKS	NOTES
Tx grp	13	12	13	Initial tx group patients
Control	12 (11 went to Crossover)	7	9	11 Crossover patients
Total	25/24	19	22	Total patients

From the paper,

> *"Eleven patients were included in the [crossover] study. Mean wound chronicity was 21.1 ± 12.4 weeks (median 19 weeks, range 11-54) and mean wound size was 4.7 ± 5.0 cm2, at baseline. Complete healing was achieved in 55% by 4 weeks, 64% by 6 weeks and 91% by 12 weeks with bi-weekly dHACM application. Mean weeks to complete healing was 4.2 ± 3.1 weeks for the 10 patients healed. After 4 weeks of standard care, wounds had decreased in size an average of 26.8 ± 45.3% versus 87.6 ± 16.0% after 4 weeks of dHACM treatment (two applications; p< 0.001)."*

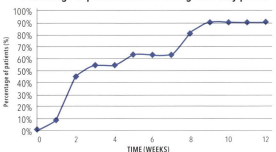

Percentage of patients healed during the study period

Figure 53. Comparison of wound surface area reduction from baseline for patients receiving the Standard of Care and for patients after the application of EpiFix.

These results collectively reflect robust product effectiveness. Compare these results to the major clinical trial that was done to evaluate Dermagraft effectiveness for DFU treatment, where out of 130 patients, 10% healed at 4 weeks; 22% healed at 8 weeks, and 30% healed at 12 weeks.[270,271] Comparison of the overall healing effects of EpiFix compared with historical clinical trials of competing products reveals a clear advantage with the use of EpiFix.

Zelen, C; Serena, T; Fetterolf, D. Dehydrated human amnion/chorion membrane allografts in patients with chronic diabetic foot ulcers: A long-term follow-up study. (Published in Wound Medicine, 2014)

In a final publication, the investigators examined the long term durability of the healing of these wounds. Investigators and clinicians from earlier case series mentioned above commented on and documented the somewhat unusual finding that the wounds closed with EpiFix remained closed long after the initial healing had occurred. In an effort to confirm that result, patients from the original and crossover populations were followed for periods of up to one year to confirm that healing created by EpiFix dHACM remained and did not recur at the same location.[81] From the article,

> *"Twenty-two patients with chronic DFU that healed with the use of dHACM were eligible for inclusion. All eligible patients had completed a single-center randomized clinical trial comparing rates of primary healing over a 12 week period with dHACM versus a standard regimen of care (Zelen et al., 2013). Follow-up examinations were scheduled for 9–12 months after primary healing with dHACM. Subsequent evaluation of clinical records was made with IRB approval and patient consent. Eighteen of 22 eligible patients (81.8%) returned for follow-up examination. Mean wound size prior to treatment with dHACM was 3.1 ± 3.8 cm², median 1.7 cm² (0.7, 13.5). Mean time to wound closure after dHACM initiation was 3.1 ± 2.8 weeks (median 2.0 weeks, range 1.0–9.0 weeks). At the 9–12 month follow-up visit 17 of 18 (94.4%) wounds treated with dHACM remained fully healed."*

Zelen, CM; Serena, TE; Snyder, RJ. A prospective, randomized comparative study of weekly versus biweekly application of dehydrated human amnion/chorion membrane allograft in the management of diabetic foot ulcers. (Published in International Wound Journal, 2014)

The optimal dosing or timing for the application of EpiFix dHACM allografts was investigated in another randomized controlled trial. Extensive reports from the medical community on the rapid healing properties in wounds treated more frequently informed the design of this trial, where weekly application of dHACM was compared with then standard biweekly application recommended for the use of the membrane. In this study, 40 patients were randomized to either weekly or biweekly applications of EpiFix dHACM (weekly n=20, biweekly n=20) in addition to non-adherent, moist dressing with compressive wrapping. Results of this comparison were statistically significant and clearly indicated that weekly application of EpiFix dHACM to diabetic foot ulcers was superior to every other week application of the material.[84]

The difference in healing rates for weekly vs. biweekly application of EpiFix dHACM is illustrated below in Figure 54 and demonstrates a clear clinical and economic preference for weekly application of the material:

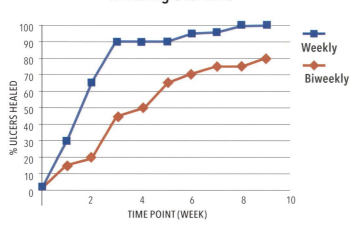

Figure 54. Rates of healing over time for each study group.

From the article,

> *"This was an institutional review board-approved, registered, prospective, randomized, comparative, non-blinded, single-center clinical trial. Patients with non-infected ulcers of ≥4 weeks duration were included for the study. They were randomized to receive weekly or biweekly application of allograft in addition to a non-adherent, moist dressing with compressive wrapping. All wounds were offloaded. The primary study outcome was mean time to healing.*
>
> *Overall, during the 12-week study period, 92.5% (37/40) ulcers completely healed. Mean time to complete healing was 4.1 ± 2.9 weeks versus 2.4 ± 1.8 weeks (p=0.039) in the biweekly versus weekly groups, respectively. Complete healing occurred in 50% versus 90% by 4 weeks in the biweekly and weekly groups, respectively (p=0.014). Number of grafts applied to healed wounds was similar at 2.4 ± 1.5 grafts and 2.3 ± 1.8 grafts for biweekly versus weekly groups, respectively (p=0.841).*
>
> *These results validate previous studies showing that the allograft is an effective treatment for diabetic ulcers and show that wounds treated with weekly application heal more rapidly than with biweekly application. More rapid healing may decrease clinical operational costs and prevent long-term medical complications."*

10.4 COMPARATIVE EFFECTIVENESS STUDY

Zelen, CM; Gould, L; Serena, TE; Carter, M.; Keller, J; Li, W. A prospective, randomised, controlled, multi-center comparative effectiveness study of healing using dehydrated human amnion/chorion membrane allograft, bioengineered skin substitute, or standard of care for treatment of chronic lower extremity diabetic ulcers. (Published in International Wound Journal, 2014)

In the next randomized controlled trial in the series, MiMedx examined the clinical cost effectiveness of EpiFix compared with a leading skin substitute product and Standard of Care in one of a very few head to head, cost effectiveness studies with these types of products.[47] The prospective multi-center randomized controlled trial (RCT) was conducted at three sites to compare the healing effectiveness of chronic lower extremity diabetic ulcers treated with either weekly applications of Apligraf, EpiFix, or standard wound care with collagen-alginate dressing.

The highlights of the study include the following key points:

- *After 4 weeks, 85% of EpiFix patients achieved complete healing compared to only 35% of Apligraf patients.*
- *After 6 weeks, 95% of EpiFix patients achieved complete healing compared to only 45% of Apligraf patients.*
- *Median time to healing with EpiFix was 13 days compared to 49 days with Apligraf.*
- *Mean number of EpiFix grafts used was 2.51 at an average cost of $1,669, compared to 6.2 Apligraf grafts used at a cost of $9,216.*
- *For every square centimeter of EpiFix wasted, approximately 61.5 square centimeters of Apligraf was wasted.*
- *EpiFix had a superior rate of wound healing and significantly faster rate of wound closure while utilizing 65% fewer grafts and 97.1% fewer square centimeters of graft material.*
- *EpiFix dramatically reduces wastage and costs while achieving superior clinical results.*

Graphically, the mean percentage of wound area healed per week showed a rapid initial increase, with progression to complete healing over time as seen in previous studies, and with more rapid and more complete healing results than when compared with either Standard of Care or Apligraf, as shown in Figure 55.

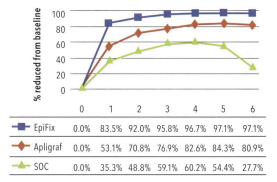

MEAN % WOUND AREA HEALED PER WEEK

	0	1	2	3	4	5	6
EpiFix	0.0%	83.5%	92.0%	95.8%	96.7%	97.1%	97.1%
Apligraf	0.0%	53.1%	70.8%	76.9%	82.6%	84.3%	80.9%
SOC	0.0%	35.3%	48.8%	59.1%	60.2%	54.4%	27.7%

Figure 55. Percent reduction in lower extremity diabetic ulcer surface area following treatment with EpiFix, compared to Organogenesis Apligraf bioengineered skin substitute and Standard of Care treatment with collagen-alginate dressing.

Looking at it another way, as the percentage of patients having complete healing at 4 and 6 weeks, we note a substantial difference between the two competing treatments as shown in Figure 56:

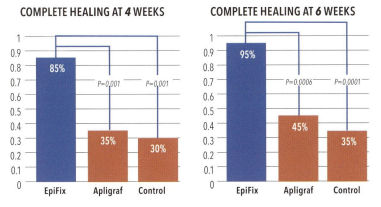

Figure 56. Percentage of patients who experienced complete healing after 4 and 6 weeks of EpiFix treatment, compared to Organogenesis Apligraf bioengineered skin substitute and Standard of Care treatment with collagen-alginate dressing.

This study also meticulously kept track of individual expenses for each of the treatment arms, and similarly, noted a substantial difference in costs between the two therapies, as shown in Figure 57:

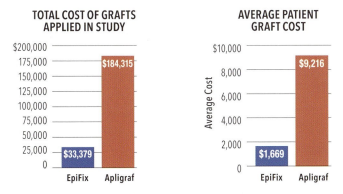

Figure 57. Cost comparison between EpiFix and Apligraf.

Note that the difference in both total costs of the grafts in the study and the average per patient graft cost in the study was significantly less expensive for EpiFix by a factor of five.

In summary, this comparative effectiveness study examining the effectiveness of EpiFix vs. a leading competing product and against Standard of Care in an IRB approved, formal clinical study reaffirms both the efficacy and cost effectiveness of the product in healing diabetic ulcers alone and in comparison with a leading skin substitute.

10.5 MULTICENTER VENOUS LEG ULCER TRIAL

Serena, TE; Carter, MJ; Le, LT; Sabo, MJ; DiMarco, DT; the EpiFix VLU Study Group. Multi-center randomized controlled clinical trial evaluating the use of dehydrated human amnion/chorion membrane allografts and multi-layer compression therapy vs. multi-layer compression therapy alone in the treatment of venous leg ulcers. (Published in Wound Repair Regeneration, 2014)

In still another randomized controlled trial for lower extremity ulcers, the effectiveness of MiMedx PURION Processed dHACM in **venous leg ulcers** was investigated using a multicenter, randomized controlled study at eight clinical sites across the United States.[93]

The purpose of this multi-center, randomized, controlled study was to evaluate the safety and efficacy of one or two applications of MiMedx dHACM and multi-layer compression therapy (MLCT) versus MLCT alone in the treatment of venous leg ulcers. The primary study outcome was proportion of patients with ≥40% reduction of wound size at 4 weeks for those receiving dHACM versus those receiving MLCT only, a surrogate endpoint found throughout the literature. Of the 84 participants enrolled in this published analysis, 53 were randomized to receive allograft and 31 were randomized to the control group. *At 4 weeks, 62% in the allograft group and 32% in the control group demonstrated a ≥40% wound closure (p=0.005) thus demonstrating a <u>significant difference between the allograft-treated groups and the multi-layer compression therapy</u> alone group at the 4-week surrogate endpoint, as shown in Figure 58. After 4 weeks wounds treated with allograft had reduced in size by a mean of 48.1% compared to 19.0% for controls, as shown in Figure 59. Venous leg ulcers treated with allograft had a significant improvement in healing at 4 weeks compared to multi-layer compression therapy alone.*

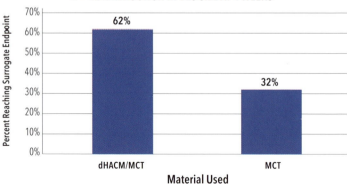

Figure 58. Reduction in wound size of ≥40% in patients receiving MiMedx dHACM and MLCT versus those receiving MLCT only; 62% versus 32%, respectively (p=0.005).

AVERAGE PERCENT REDUCTION IN SIZE

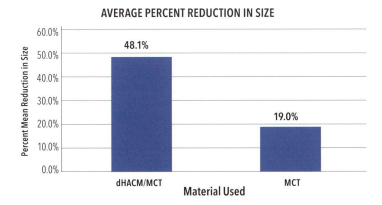

Figure 59. After 4 weeks mean reductions of 48.1% for EpiFix patients versus 19.0% for MLCT only patients were observed (p=0.005).

Percent of wound reduction was similar for those receiving 1 or 2 dHACM applications at 51.9% and 44.4% respectively, as shown in Figure 60. (The investigators speculate that wider separation of these dose administration curves, as was observed above with diabetic foot ulcers, might occur at longer time periods. The difference with more aggressive frequency of dosing and over a longer follow up period is being evaluated in the next multicenter VLU study as outlined below.)

MEAN PERCENT REDUCTION IN WOUND SIZE

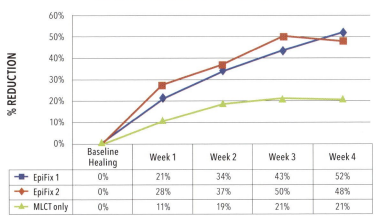

	Baseline Healing	Week 1	Week 2	Week 3	Week 4
EpiFix 1	0%	21%	34%	43%	52%
EpiFix 2	0%	28%	37%	50%	48%
MLCT only	0%	11%	19%	21%	21%

Figure 60. Mean percent reduction in wound size during the 4 week study period.

Within the EpiFix dHACM group, wound area was reduced by a mean of 2.28 ± 3.04 cm^2 during the study period (from randomization to end of study). For those patients receiving MLCT only, wound area was not reduced as much during the study period with a mean difference of only 0.41 ± 2.68 cm^2 between randomization and the 4-week visit. In the 4-week study period, 6 patients in the dHACM group and 4 patients in the MLCT group had complete wound closure.

Pain scores were also collected at randomization and week 4 for 49 patients in the dHACM group and 28 patients in the MLCT only group using a visual analogue scale (VAS). Of those with recorded pain scores (44/49 [89.8%]) in the dHACM group reported VLU pain at randomization and in the MLCT group (21/28 [75.0%]) reported VLU pain. During the study period 35/44 (79.5%) of patients in the dHACM group reported a reduction in pain from the randomization visit when dHACM was applied and the 4-week visit, as shown in Figure 61. For patients receiving MLCT only, 11/21 (52.4%) reported reduced VLU pain in the study period.

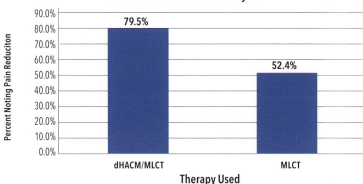

Figure 61. Pain reduction was observed to be greater for the dHACM study group with 79.5% of patients reporting pain reduction versus 52.4% of patients in the MLCT group.

The results of this multi-center randomized clinical trial show that VLUs treated with dHACM and MLCT experience an accelerated rate of healing compared with VLUs treated with MLCT alone. These results demonstrate that the addition of dHACM to MCT is more efficacious for the treatment of VLUs.

10.6 COMPARATIVE BENCHMARK STUDY

In summary, robust results of clinical efficacy have been demonstrated now **in more than 300 clinical trial patients** across various studies, where consistent, significant outcomes have been observed. Even in the smaller, initial clinical trials, statistical power is sufficient to conclude a positive outcome. Small numbers are able to demonstrate a positive and significant conclusion because of the large effect sizes observed.

The above findings, while notable in themselves, are further underscored by comparing related clinical trial findings from existing medical literature on comparable competitive products. In this regard, MiMedx recently published the results of a detailed literature analysis of published studies containing information on the effectiveness of several advanced wound care products.[92] Data from this analysis indicate that complete wound closure within 12 weeks of treatment initiation occurred in 56%, 30%, and 92% of Apligraf, Dermagraft, and EpiFix-treated diabetic foot ulcers, respectively, as shown in Figure 62. EpiFix-treated diabetic foot ulcers had the shortest time to healing (median 14 days) and least amount of graft material used (14 cm²) versus comparative products in the studies examined. Rate of ulcer recurrence was 5.9% for Apligraf (after 6 months), 18.8% for Dermagraft (after 8 months), and 5.6% for EpiFix (after 9–12 months).[92] The following collected information in Table XII presents a comparative analysis and contextually frames the healing ability of the EpiFix allograft in a larger pooled sample group.

Table XII. Wound area and healing metrics as reported in randomized controlled trials.[80,81,83,84,270,272]

	Apligraf (n=112)	Dermagraft (n=130)	EpiFix (n=64)
Wound area (cm²)	2.97 ± 3.10	2.31	2.72 ± 2.6
Mean grafts received*	3.9	5.7	2.4
Complete wound closure within 12 weeks	56% 63/112	30% 39/130	92% 59/64
Median days to closure	65 (7, 88) (n=63)	NR	14 (7, 77) (n=59)
Ulcer recurrence	5.9%[1]	18.8%[2]	5.6%[3]
Adverse events** (infection, cellulitis, osteomyelitis)	22.3%	19%	1.6%

Data reported as mean ± SD, percentage, or median (min, max) as indicated.
[1]At 6 months. [2]At 8 months (32 weeks). [3]At 9-12 months.
* To healing or to maximum allowed during 12 week study period
** Of study wound

From the article,

"For each product evaluated, the definition of complete wound healing was defined as full epithelialization of the wound with the absence of drainage. Healing rates at 6, 9, and 12 weeks are presented in Figure [62]. Of the products evaluated, wounds treated with EpiFix had the highest rate of complete closure (92%) at the end of the 12-week study period, compared with a 56% closure rate with Apligraf and a 30% closure rate with Dermagraft (all pairwise comparisons p<0.001). Within 6 weeks of the first graft application, 81% of ulcers treated with EpiFix were closed versus 35% and 15% of Apligraf- and Dermagraft-treated wounds, respectively (all pairwise comparisons p≤0.003)."

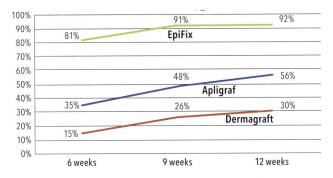

Figure 62. Rates of complete healing for Apligraf, Dermagraft, and EpiFix groups.

As noted above, the research quantifies the improved time to healing with the EpiFix allografts over the other competing products. Notably, this study also noted the decreased numbers of grafts needed to resolve wounds on average when comparing EpiFix to the other grafts, as shown in Figures 63 and 64. This in turn translates into a substantial cost savings that can readily be measured or modelled, as shown in Figure 65.

COMPARISON OF QUANTITY AND ESTIMATED COST OF PRODUCTS USED PER PATIENT:

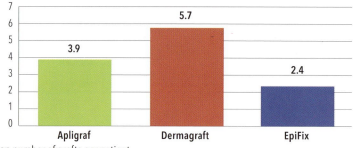

Figure 63. Mean number of grafts per patient.

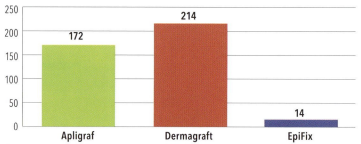

Figure 64. Total product used per patient (sq cm).

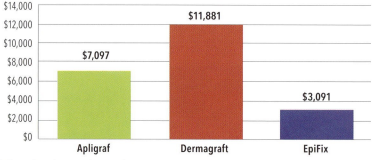

Figure 65. Cost of product used per patient.

With fewer grafts, and a more focused cost structure due to multiple available sizes, the EpiFix allografts clearly separate themselves from the two to almost four times as expensive Dermagraft or Apligraf alternatives.

Finally, this article also reviewed the relative safety and durability of each of these products. Percent of serious wound complications were lowest with EpiFix when compared across all three products, and the durability of the EpiFix regenerative effects on the integumentary system are robust with time.

10.7 STATISTICAL INFERENCE IN MIMEDX CLINICAL TRIALS

The clinical trials described in this document are each memorable and significant for the dramatic effect size seen when using dHACM in a clinical setting, either in a case series or in formal randomized clinical trials. As noted above, the robust nature of this effect size is seen across different investigators, across different geographic regions and even in different disease states or conditions.

These observations support and corroborate the findings in each of these trials, despite what has been criticized as a smaller number of patients. The dramatic effectiveness of dHACM used in clinical studies obviates the need for the large clinical trials necessary to compare earlier "last generation" biologic materials against Standard of Care, where the effect size, while statistically significant, was much smaller. The MiMedx clinical trials are in fact both appropriately powered and statistically significant to form conclusions about the effectiveness of the allografts. One might consider the converse situation, where application of a material causes an immediate adverse reaction or death in the test individual in all situations where it is used. Clinical trials begun with such materials would also be small indeed, yet would still be statistically valid and provide sufficient information to form conclusions.

When clinical trials are conducted, one of the jobs of the statistician is to figure out how many subjects have to be enrolled. This is done through sample size calculations with sophisticated software (e.g., PASS 11). In general, the *power* of the primary endpoint of the trial (and sometimes the trial's secondary endpoints) is targeted to be between 80 and 90%. Power is the likelihood that a study will detect an effect, if an effect truly exists in the population.

The number of subjects needed to reach a given power for an endpoint is highly dependent (among other things) on the effect size, which is a measure of the strength of a treatment—efficacy if it is a controlled trial and effectiveness if it is a pragmatic non-controlled trial. So, for example, if at 12 weeks the proportion of wounds healed in the control group (standard or usual care) was 30% but the proportion of wounds healed in the treatment group was 90%, one would know that they are dealing with a relatively large effect size. Conversely, if the proportion of wounds healed in the treatment group had been 40%, then the additional 10% of healed wounds, which the treatment conferred, would mean a relatively small effect size. While statisticians use a number of different ways to estimate effect size, MiMedx uses Cohen's *d* to calculate the effect size in several examples for continuous variables (such a surface area reduction), and *phi*, for cross-tabulations, such as those used in *chi* square (2x2 contingency tables), which are applicable to proportions of wound healed. A Cohen's *d* value of 0.2 would signify a small effect size, 0.5 a medium effect size, and 0.8 a large effect size while the corresponding figures for φ would be 0.1, 0.3, and 0.5. All things being equal, when the effect size of the treatment to be tested is large, a much smaller number of subjects (or wounds) is required in the trial. Commonly, many wound care trials are criticized as having too small a sample size for the demonstrated effect size. Another way of saying this is that the trial was underpowered to stand a reasonable chance of detecting significant results in given endpoints.

Whether to conduct interim analyses of a clinical trial while recruitment continues is still a matter of debate. Those opposed to interim analysis say that it is a waste of time unless one acts upon the results, and that in most cases it will not make a difference. Of course, there are those who beg to differ. The simplest form of trial monitoring is to recalculate the sample size based on the required power for one or more endpoints. In the trial protocol this is specified at various points in the trial based on the percentage of subjects who have completed the study. This approach avoids so-called *alpha* penalties because one is not actually analyzing the results, and at the same time provides a rough measure of whether assumptions are holding up. Also, it is only worth doing interim analyses if the trial has a relatively large number of subjects or recruitment is likely to be very slow. Typically the first interim results indicate whether prior assumptions before the trial started are more or less right, were overly optimistic, or pessimistic. In the first instance, the trial continues as planned; in the second instance there is the possibility to end the trial with fewer subjects provided all the results of all the important endpoints look good. This can potentially lower the overall costs of the trial and reduce patient exposure to risks (the equipoise issue: equipoise provides the ethical basis for medical research that involves assigning patients to different treatment arms of a clinical trial). The third scenario is obviously not welcome, but gives the sponsor the chance to terminate the trial early if the chances of completing it are slim (too many subjects required), thus saving money and improving equipoise. This overall approach can also satisfy trial stakeholders to assure them that the trial is either providing expected results or that a sponsor has taken some appropriate steps to halt a poor trial. More formal group sequential analyses can be undertaken. In this method, a mathematical simulation is undertaken to calculate the penalties for statistical significance based on the number of times an actual statistical analysis of an endpoint is undertaken while the trial is running and the means of apportioning the penalty (increasing with time, equal, etc.). This kind of analysis is more common in larger trials in which the effect size tends to be much smaller.

The population that is analyzed is also important. In controlled trials, especially randomized controlled trials (RCTs), it is important to first analyze all subjects that took part in the trial regardless of outcome, whether the subject was withdrawn from the trial, or even died during the trial. This is called an "intention to treat" (ITT) analysis. Another commonly analyzed population includes per protocol, which simply means that only those subjects who had no clinical trial protocol violations are included in the analysis. When the RCT does not have an ITT analysis in a published journal article, it is likely that something went wrong in the trial, or the treatment did not perform as expected; often the effect size was much smaller than anticipated.

Some clinical trials are conducted at a single site and some using many sites (multi-site trials). In general, multi-site trials are preferable because they tell much about the heterogeneity of trial practice. However, if this heterogeneity is high it can lead to analysis problems. A single site will often provide cleaner endpoint results, which is particularly useful in a controlled trial to understand effect size, but a single site may or may not be representative, regardless of whether it is a controlled trial or not.

EpiFix Clinical Trials

EpiFix is an amniotic membrane wound graft developed by MiMedx that is used as an adjunct treatment in chronic wounds. In order to demonstrate its efficacy, that is, how effective EpiFix is under controlled conditions, MiMedx sponsored a number of clinical trials that involved subjects with diabetic foot ulcers.

Randomized Controlled Trial Comparing EpiFix to Standard of Care (Diabetic Foot Ulcers)

In this trial,[80] subjects were randomized to Standard of Care (SOC), comprising debridement, moist wound care therapy, and offloading (removable cast walker), or SOC plus application of EpiFix every 2 weeks.

The sample size of the trial was very small (SOC: 12; EpiFix: 13) but the ITT results are impressive: at 4 weeks 10/13 subjects had completely healed compared to 0/12 SOC subjects ($p < 0.001$) and the mean wound surface area reduction was 32.0% for the SOC group vs. 97.1% for the EpiFix group ($p<0.001$). At 6 weeks, the figures were 12/13 (92%) vs. 1/12 (8%), and –1.8% vs. 98.4% (both p values <0.001). respectively. The statistical tests used to analyze the probabilities of attaining these results were appropriate (*chi square and Mann–Whitney U test*), and the absolute p values were recalculated at about 0.0001. Although no specific adjustment of the familywise error rate (FWER) was undertaken, using the most conservative approach—the full Bonferroni correction, which would result in the level of statistical significance being set at 0.0125—all results still remain very statistically significant. While sample size calculations are not mentioned in the text of the published study, calculations were undertaken prior to start of the trial. A post-hoc analysis conducted using Pass 11 (PASS 11 is software for estimating the number of subjects that should be used in a study through statistical power analysis) shows that power was 98-100% depending on the test used with *alpha* set to 0.0125. Calculated Cohen's *d* values were 1.9-2.0 and φ values were 0.78-0.84, indicating very large effect sizes. Consequently, even though N for the trial is very small, and replication desirable, the study was large enough to demonstrate very statistically significant results in terms of the efficacy of EpiFix to speed healing in chronic diabetic foot ulcers.

Subject and wound characteristic differences between the groups were small and would not have affected the overall results. Other covariates not reported would also have been unlikely to affect the results as well.

An additional piece of evidence is the crossover trial,[83] in which the 11 subjects whose wounds had not healed in the original RCT,[80] were given EpiFix in the same manner as for the RCT. At 6 weeks 7/11 wounds had healed and by 12 weeks, 10/11 wounds had healed. It can be argued that although the wound trajectory was not quite as fast as seen in those subjects from the EpiFix arm of the RCT, the vast majority of these recalcitrant wounds nevertheless did heal.

Finally, a long-term follow-up of subjects in the RCT demonstrated that 94% (17/18 patients that could be followed up) still had fully healed diabetic foot ulcers.[81] The corollary of this result—the incidence of ulcer recurrence, which is 5-6%—is much lower than one might have expected. While these are small numbers and it is possible that these subjects might be considered relatively healthy, which could lower ulcer recurrence, it is also possible that EpiFix might have some relatively longer-term benefits that need to be better understood.

Randomized Controlled Trial Comparing Different Frequencies of EpiFix Application (Diabetic Foot Ulcers)

In this RCT,[84] different application rates of EpiFix were tested to determine whether more frequent applications would further improve the wound trajectory. Both groups received SOC while 1 group had weekly application of EpiFix compared to an application every 2 weeks, per the first RCT.[80] Otherwise the trial was conducted similarly to the first RCT with appropriate statistics tests employed.

Again the sample size was small (20 in each group) but the results showed evidence that more frequent application of EpiFix sped up healing compared to application every 2 weeks. Primary endpoint was mean time to heal, with 8 other secondary endpoints. In all instances, wounds healed faster in the weekly group at each point in time compared to the every 2 weeks group. Again, no adjustment for the FWER was made, so in this instance the Hochberg set-up procedure was employed, which is technically a false discovery rate (FDR) procedure, slightly less stringent than the FWER full Bonferroni correction. The adjusted *p* values (only including wound healing endpoints) showed that 3 endpoints were statistically significant: wound size at week 2 (*p*=0.006; every other week: mean wound area, 0.91 cm²; weekly: 0.09 cm²); completely healed by week 2 (*p*=0.036; every other week: 4/20; weekly: 13/20); and completely healed by week 4 (*p*=0.037; every other week: 10/20; weekly: 18/20). Post-hoc calculated power values were 84% for the 2 statistically significant proportion of healed wounds and 76% for the comparison of wound area. Effect sizes were obviously not as large as in the first RCT but were still respectable: Cohen's d value was 0.82 and φ values were between 0.44 and 0.46, indicating a medium to large effect size obtained by doubling the frequency of EpiFix application.

Although it can be argued that a more judicious analytical plan might have improved the *p* values for key wound-healing endpoints, the present analysis still shows that the effect size is not trivial, that power in most instances was reasonable or close to reasonable, and that there are statistically significant differences favoring faster healing of chronic DFUs when EpiFix is applied weekly instead of every other week.

Randomized Controlled Trial Comparing Different Frequencies of EpiFix Application (Venous Leg Ulcers)

This controlled trial[93] was similar in the dosing regimen to the dosage trial treating chronic DFUs but differed in one major respect: surrogate endpoints were employed rather than a complete wound healing endpoint. The use of surrogate endpoints is still a controversial topic in wound care, in part because validation to date has shown that overall accuracy (technically the receiver operating characteristic) is not as high as one would like it. For example, the large study conducted by Gelfand et al[273] showed a receiver operating characteristic (ROC) of 0.76 (76%) when the percentage reduction in wound area at 4 weeks was used to predict complete wound healing at 24 weeks; this is somewhere between "acceptable" and "good." However, compared to other medical specialties, wound care has had traditionally only one clearly meaningful hard endpoint—complete wound healing—and that end point as currently defined by the FDA can be problematic for many situations.[274] Several wound care groups are now starting to address this (and other issues) with the FDA but it may be some time before compromise is reached.

Accepting the fact that surrogate endpoints have some limitations, the trial clearly showed that a significantly higher proportion of patients with chronic VLUs treated with EpiFix (1 or 2 treatments) and multilayer compression therapy for 4 weeks reached 40% closure compared to subjects whose VLUs were just treated with multilayer compression therapy (62% vs. 32%; *p*=0.005). This result reflects the mean reduction in VLU area over the 4-week period of 48.1% vs. 19.0% for these groups. In respect of dosage, the result obtained with 1 application of EpiFix was almost identical with that obtained with 2 doses (pieces): 62% vs. 63%. Post-hoc calculated power value was 77% for the primary surrogate endpoint, which is close to the minimum of 80% recommended for endpoints, and effect size (φ value) was 0.29, which is a medium effect.

There has been some criticism of this trial in the literature, and the authors have replied to address the points raised. While no wound care trials have been perfectly designed or conducted (If one knew how wound care trials would turn out, one would not be doing research!), and there were some limitations to this particular trial, the end result is that EpiFix had a substantial and statistically significant effect on the healing of VLUs early in the wound healing trajectory that would enable many wounds to be healed that might have otherwise taken a very long time to heal.

A majority of subjects in this trial have been followed over a longer period of time and analysis is in progress to determine healing over this longer period of time.

Randomized Controlled Trial Comparing EpiFix to Apligraf and Standard of Care (Diabetic Foot Ulcers)

In this controlled trial there were 3 arms to which subjects were randomly allocated after excluding subjects whose wounds had decreased in area by more than 20% during the 2-week run-in period: SOC (Standard of Care), SOC + EpiFix or SOC + Apligraf.[47] SOC included wound cleansing, debridement (if appropriate), moist wound care, and offloading (cast walker), and EpiFix or Apligraf was applied weekly for a maximum of 6 weeks. At 6 weeks 95% of subjects treated with EpiFix had healed compared to 45% of Apligraf-treated subjects and 35% of subjects treated with SOC alone. These results were statistically significant: EpiFix vs. Apligraf (p=0.0006); EpiFix vs. SOC (p=0.0001). Despite the relatively small sample sizes (20 in each group), the Hochberg-adjusted p values clearly reflected a large effect size (φ) of 0.55-0.63, depending on which group was compared to the EpiFix group. Post-hoc analysis shows an achieved power in this statistical analysis of 97-99.6%, which is outstanding. Kaplan-Meier analysis, a type of survival analysis, also showed that median time to heal was 13 days for the EpiFix group and 49 days for the other groups (p<0.0001, Hochberg-adjusted).

While critics might say that the trial was not conducted for the usual length of time in wound care studies (e.g., 12 weeks), or that sample sizes were too small, the results speak for themselves in that by 6 weeks the vast majority of DFUs treated with EpiFix were healed. This is a classic example of demonstrating that when large effect sizes are present in a treatment group, one does not need large sample sizes nor long periods of treatment to reach a conclusion.

A simple health economics analysis was also performed based on the results of the trial, which showed that use of EpiFix was vastly cheaper to heal a wound compared to Apligraf ($9,216 vs. $1,669 per patient). This is an example of cost minimization analysis and does not take into account any costs associated with the visit, Standard of Care, or any other treatments.

138

10.8 OTHER "COMPARATIVE STUDIES" FROM THE LITERATURE

Recently, a number of retrospective clinical studies have reached the literature comparing EpiFix with other biologic wound therapies that suggest different outcomes than those mentioned above, and/or with the suggestion that other often competing products may be superior. A review of a few of these articles and the limitations of their approach is instructive.

10.8.1 ORGANOGENESIS APLIGRAF® ARTICLE

A recent publication funded by Organogenesis is entitled *"Comparative Effectiveness of a Bioengineered Living Cellular Construct vs. a Dehydrated Human Amniotic Membrane Allograft for the Treatment of Diabetic Foot Ulcers in a Real World Setting"* by Kirsner et al.[275] This retrospective analysis of data collected in an electronic medical record, seeks to compare the effectiveness of dehydrated human amnion/chorion membrane (EpiFix) allograft in comparison to their product Apligraf.

Comparative effectiveness research aims to compare various therapies in a manner that establishes the effectiveness of one therapy over another. It would seem to be straightforward. If two therapies are equally priced, one would chose the more effective one. If two therapies are equivalent (or one is at least "noninferior" to the other), if all things were equal, one would select the cheaper one. If a simple decision were not easy to discern, then one might compare data points on a chart to make a decision with the best trade off in value and cost.

Papers such as the one referred to in this section however, inject a commercial bias that is unhelpful towards meeting this goal. While the authors claim that the data provide a snap shot of "real world" effectiveness of Apligraf and EpiFix, the approach taken does not consistently control for the very complex environmental factors in the "real world" that makes such a comparison impossible in such an unstructured approach.

The data used are extracted from an electronic medical record (EMR) system. The authors would have been better served to more clearly describe the ability of the data to accurately represent a real world environment. EMR input is often not of the robust consistent accuracy that formal research data collection must follow, is not audited, and may have gaps or inaccuracies, particularly where practice patterns are established. For example, in "real" real world data the average size of a DFU billed through Centers for Medicare & Medicaid Services (CMS) is 1.35 sq cm. In this article, it appears the sizes that were "selected" were 6 sq cm and 5.2 sq cm-- which are inconsistent with CMS and other numbers.[276,277]

The accepted standard for making comparative superiority claims is the prospective, randomized, properly evaluated clinical trial. Unfortunately for these authors, valid, scientifically rigorous studies come to a different conclusion than they do.

Evidence prepared from a randomized controlled clinical trial supported by MiMedx with an independent investigator described above concludes that the EpiFix allografts are superior to Apligraf, not the other way around. In those studies, patient populations are selected for consistency, properly randomized, and treated in a manner that the only variable is the placement of the EpiFix allograft or Apligraf material.

This information is further complemented by analyses of the published, peer reviewed literature and studies that are more robust. Such a comparison using the existing published data from the company's actual trials also supports a different conclusion than that presented in the paper.[92]

The use of medical informatics here to create a comparative analysis seems to have been prepared without proper controls, in a biased environment, and with results that contradict the rest of the medical literature. In an effort to promote a particular product, it may succeed, but as presenting a legitimate piece of scientific research, it fails on numerous counts.

10.8.2 ALLIQUA BIOVANCE® COMPARISON ARTICLE

The journal *Wounds* recently published an article titled, "Real-world Experience With a Decellularized Dehydrated Human Amniotic Membrane Allograft" that ostensibly provided validation for the use of a particular brand of amniotic membrane allograft in multiple clinical situations.[278] It purports to present a valid "registry," from which data were extracted and analyzed.[278] This is actually a simple review of a selection of 10 year old cases in a spreadsheet.

A number of plainly apparent methodological flaws are noted. For example, this is not a registry study. Rather, what is reported here is an open label surveillance or simple trial whose results were transcribed to a spreadsheet. Other elements of structure are similarly lacking. For example, the relatively small numbers of patients reviewed for this time period across a number of sites and with a number of underlying etiologies would strongly suggest this is a selected group.

This "study" consisted of 2 observation points – clinical data collected at the "baseline" and last visit. There are no data to assess safety and effectiveness, wound care techniques, etc., for intervening visits. Photographs were taken, but no further mention is made of them. Whether the materials and methods section were reviewed by an IRB or were granted an IRB exemption was also not specified. This is all not consistent with a robust study.

As another example, the authors note that "this study was observational; there was neither treatment randomization nor blinding, and there were no control groups." Without controls the observations are virtually meaningless. Most true registries will have a reference group control, even if the observations are not blinded.

The clinical conditions were varied – DFU, VLU, ischemic vascular, and autoimmune vasculitic wounds – diversity that makes estimates of effectiveness, particularly on a "first visit to last visit" assessment almost meaningless. Each of these wound types have their own underlying issues, different approaches, co-morbidities, etc. Granted, the authors point out that randomized controlled trials typically have inclusion and exclusion criteria that reduce the heterogeneity of the patient population under study to create a homogeneous group that can be used to evaluate a therapy against controls. Results collected in this latter way are scientifically meaningless, as they are here.

The "data" were then sent to the sponsor and entered into Excel spreadsheets for analysis and included categorical data, numbers, and notes in comment fields. This is not an interactive database such as those commonly deployed for statistical analysis of clinical results.

Regarding study limitations, the authors noted: "The study did not have a control arm nor were the wound measurements provided at regular intervals, but were done only on enrollment and at the end of the study. Therefore, it is difficult to determine how the application of DDHAM [decellularized dehydrated human amniotic membrane] compares to other treatment regimens with respect to wound closure outcomes. In addition, the average period during which subjects participated was shorter than in most studies." In all, there are in fact a number of limitations that come from the fact that the authors are not consistent with the current methods, analytic elements, and guidelines for evaluating wound care cases well known to the readership of this journal.

The smaller number of actual cases involved for this series would suggest that they were somehow selected through a mechanism which is not described. (15 wound centers supplied only 165 cases.) This is further underscored by reports of the average wound sizes, which are not consistent with what is experienced in the field or with a _**real**_ "real-world" registry analysis done recently by Wilcox.[276] Noteworthy is that 50-58% of wounds did not close over roughly 10 weeks; not encouraging efficacy when other therapies and even other amniotic membrane products do better.[47]

There were a number of other procedural irregularities which should also be of concern: for example, the study data were collected in 2005, over 10 years ago. Much has changed in the treatment of wounds generally, and in the understanding and use of allografts in particular. Why publish them now? At this point it would be virtually impossible to track these patients or confirm results.

In summary, the true standard for evaluating wound care is through Level I evidence, using randomized controlled trials that systematically review the efficacy and safety of a product. Multiple examples of this approach exist in wound care and have been evaluated by the editorial staff in past issues, and guidelines exist for this type of analysis in multiple places.[274]

10.9 ONGOING RESEARCH

The original successes documented with the case reports, case series, and randomized controlled trials has led to further development and initiation of several larger, multicenter randomized controlled trials to both confirm the earlier work and demonstrate these findings in dispersed, multicenter environments. While earlier results were highly statistically significant due in large part to the dramatic effects on rate of healing, larger multicenter trials were deemed necessary to complete a comprehensive confirmation of the products applicability to general populations.

Multicenter Randomized Controlled Trial - Diabetic Leg Ulcers III

A large, multicenter, randomized controlled trial is underway, and is now being expanded across a number of sites for the treatment of lower extremity diabetic ulcers. MiMedx anticipates that formal results and publication of these findings will be available within the next year.

Multicenter Randomized Controlled Trial - Venous Leg Ulcers II

Another large, multicenter, randomized controlled trial is also currently underway for the treatment of lower extremity venous leg ulcers in patients in Department of Veterans Affairs Medical Centers, with the first of these centers now enrolling patients. Preliminary results are not yet available, but are anticipated within the next one to two years.

10.10 DOCUMENTATION OF THE CLINICAL EFFECTIVENESS OF dHACM IN WOUNDS AND OTHER APPLICATIONS

Articles Published in the Peer Reviewed Literature

Amniotic membrane prepared using the MiMedx PURION Process has found application in numerous other clinical applications in additions to wounds. A full listing of peer reviewed, clinical articles on the medical application of PURION Processed dHACM is included in **Appendix A**. Scientific articles are also included. This complements a much larger literature on the general healing properties and medical uses of amniotic membrane in general.

National Meeting Poster Presentations

Multiple reports from the field have resulted in clinicians preparing their own case histories and case series for review at national conferences and meetings. Posters presented, along with topics addressed, are included in **Appendix B**. The wide range of application possibilities and the effectiveness of dHACM as a healing medium are repeatedly demonstrated in these posters, which typically also include a peer review process as well. A number of these posters have received presentation honors. Typical types of wounds described in these poster sessions include diabetic leg ulcers, venous leg ulcers, burns, decubitus pressure ulcers, and plastic surgery applications.

Micronized dHACM in an Injectable form: Randomized Controlled Trial (RCT) of Micronized dHACM in Plantar Fasciitis (Published in Foot & Ankle International, 2013)

A powdered, micronized form of PURION Processed AmnioFix dHACM has been employed in the treatment of plantar fasciitis. Micronized AmnioFix dHACM has been proposed as an injectable treatment for various soft tissue inflammatory states where the rich supply of growth factors and cytokines present in dHACM would have a beneficial effect to enhance healing.

Results from a randomized, blinded clinical trial examining the efficacy of micronized AmnioFix dHACM in plantar fasciitis have been published.[82] Findings from this study suggest that the injection of micronized amniotic membrane in patients with refractory plantar fasciitis shows potential in reducing pain and improving the quality of life in these patients. Heel/ankle pain was significantly reduced in patients treated with these injections, as shown in Figure 66:

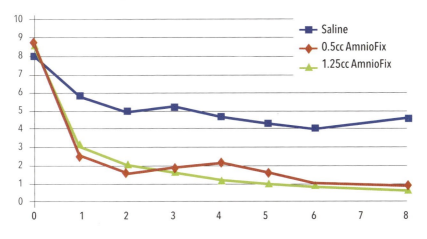

Figure 66. Wong-Baker FACES pain scores for patients in the study demonstrated decreased pain in the treatment groups over saline controls.

Similarly, improvements were observed in a commonly used, validated ankle score, as shown in Figure 67:

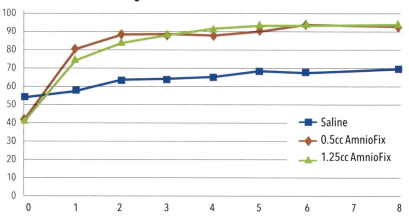

Figure 67. AOFAS Ankle – Hindfoot scores for patients in the study started out at a lower level than controls, and despite this fact, the treatment group experienced a dramatic improvement in symptoms (p<0.001).

The results of this clinical trial are being expanded in a larger, multicenter, randomized controlled trial currently underway as part of a formal Investigational New Drug (IND) application designed to develop additional strong clinical evidence for the effectiveness of this product in this indication.

Spine Surgery

AmnioFix, a derivative preparation of dHACM in which the epithelial layer is disrupted on the amnion layer of the amnion/chorion membrane, is used widely in a number of internal procedures in orthopedics and neurosurgery as an allograft to reduce the formation of scar tissue, modulate inflammation, and to enhance healing. In a clinical trial at the Virginia Spine Institute, spine surgery patients treated with AmnioFix were noted to have less scarring in the inter-fascial planes on reoperation. These findings were evident when patients were operated on for removal of previously placed segmental posterior lumbar instrumentation. This case series was recently published in *Advances in Orthopedics*.[94]

Otorhinolaryngology (Published in Otolaryngology - Head and Neck Surgery, 2014)

The application of amniotic membrane in the repair of damaged tympanic membranes was recently published by Dr. Griffith Hsu. In this paper, amniotic membrane was successfully used as an adjunctive measure to facilitate healing of perforated or damage tympanic membranes.[90]

Clinical Trials Underway in Potential Applications Other than Wounds

Several other clinical trials are currently starting that employ the use of dHACM in other potentially applicable clinical healing environments. These include:

- Randomized controlled multicenter trial testing the applicability of AmnioFix dHACM in open craniectomy procedures.
- Randomized controlled trial in a single center for confirmation of reduced scarring in patients undergoing laminectomy surgery.
- Randomized controlled trial testing the applicability of AmnioFix dHACM in nerve preservation surgery using robotic assisted (DaVinci) surgery of the prostate in patients with prostate cancer, to improve erectile dysfunction and other post-operative complications.

10.11 RESEARCH INCLUDING ECONOMIC ANALYSIS AND REVIEW OF THE PRODUCT

Economic Analysis and Review

Initial clinical work also focused on the economics of using EpiFix allografts. Early experience with various wound types led to the development of a range of EpiFix dHACM allograft sizes and configurations to better correlate with the range of sizes seen in advanced wound care practice. These efforts by the company have created a product range that has successfully reduced the overall cost of wound healing in patients in whom biological dressings are used – an outcome that marries the unmatched effectiveness of the allografts with reduced wastage.

Comparative studies using typical formulations and application regimens from competing products support the observation that EpiFix represents a truly cost competitive material, based on the reduced clinical costs of fewer applications, more efficient allograft sizes, and the longer term durability of the wound healing that occurs. Substantial documentation in this regard is available on request.[279]

10.12 CONCLUSION

Amniotic membrane has been known to have biological activity and the potential for a large number of medical applications for over a century. The underlying mechanism of this activity includes the presence of potent regenerative growth factors, cytokines, chemokines, TIMPs, and other important molecules distributed within the tissue to provide a balanced adjunctive support in a variety of healing environments. These biologically active compounds provide a direct stimulation to the healing process, including the local effects on cell differentiation, cell migration, and the cytotropic effect on mesenchymal and regional stem cells, acting as a **"stem cell magnet"** to not only create an environment for healing but draw in and engage these cells to enhance the healing process as well.

MiMedx's PURION Process, developed to successfully preserve these key biological molecules and their activity, has now created a preserved form of amniotic membrane as EpiFix and AmnioFix dHACM that has widespread clinical application and demonstrated usefulness.

With the publication of multiple randomized, multicenter controlled trials and the support of observational and case studies, the clinical effectiveness of dHACM has been firmly established. Statistically significant data from these studies have confirmed that the well-known healing properties of this material persist in the multilayer, PURION Processed MiMedx allografts. Clinical and economic evidence clearly supports the advantages these products offer physicians, patients, and payers.

Ongoing clinical research efforts have been designed to further confirm the unique properties of the EpiFix and AmnioFix dHACM material. Data from these trials will provide further support for the unique attributes of these products in addressing significant, life-altering diseases.

APPENDIX A: JOURNAL ARTICLES ON MIMEDX dHACM ALLOGRAFTS

MiMedx Articles

Chi, CS; Andrade, DB; Kimm SG; Solomon CS. "Guided Tissue Regeneration in Endodontic Surgery by Using a Bioactive Resorbable Membrane." Journal of Endodontics. 2015;41(4):559-62.

Chua, W. "Dehydrated Human Amnion/Chorion Membrane for the Treatment of Full-Thickness Plantar Burn in a Diabetic Patient: A Case Report." Journal of Diabetic Foot Complications. 2014;6(3):67-71.

Chuck, RS; Graff, JM; Bryant, MR; Sweet, PM "Biomechanical Characterization of Human Amniotic Membrane Preparations for Ocular Surface Reconstruction." Ophthalmic Research. 2004;36(6):341-348.

Fenner, A. "Amniotic Membrane Nerve Wrap Improves Continence and Potency Outcomes After Robotic Prostatectomy." Nature Reviews Urology. 2015;12(3):126.

Fetterolf, D; Savage, R. "Dehydrated Human Amniotic Tissue Improves Healing Time, Cost of Care." Today's Wound Clinic. 2013;7(1):19-20.

Fetterolf, D; Snyder, R. "Scientific and Clinical Support for the Use of Dehydrated Amniotic Membrane in Wound Management." WOUNDS. 2012;24(10):299-307.

Fetterolf, D; Istwan, N; Stanziano, G. "An Evaluation of Healing Metrics Associated With Commonly Used Advanced Wound Care Products For the Treatment of Chronic Diabetic Foot Ulcers." Managed Care. 2014;(23)7:31-38.

Forbes, J; Fetterolf, D. "Dehydrated Amniotic Membrane Allografts for the Treatment of Chronic Wounds: A Case Series." Journal of Wound Care. 2012;(21)6: 290 - 296.

Fournier, J; McLachlan, D. "Ocular Surface Reconstruction Using Amniotic Membrane Allograft for Severe Surface Disorders in Chemical Burns: Case Report and Review of the Literature." International Surgery. 2005;90(1):45-47.

Gurinsky, B. "A Novel Dehydrated Amnion Allograft for use in the Treatment of Gingival Recession: An Observational Case Series." Journal of Implant & Advanced Clinical Dentistry. 2009;1(1):65-73.

Holtzclaw, D. "Extraction Site Preservation Using New Graft Material That Combines Mineralized and Demineralized Allograft Bone: A Case Series Report with Histology." Compendium of Continuing Education in Dentistry. 2014;35(2):107-112.

Holtzclaw, D. "Open Sinus Lift Healing Comparison Between a Non-Perforated Schneiderian Membrane and a Perforated Schneiderian Membrane Repaired with Amnion-Chorion Allograft Barrier: A Controlled Split Mouth Case Report." Journal of Implant & Advanced Clinical Dentistry. 2014;6(8): 11-21.

Holtzclaw, D; Toscano, N "Amnion Chorion Allograft Barrier: Indications and Techniques Update." Journal of Implant & Advanced Clinical Dentistry. 2011;4(2):25-38.

Holtzclaw, D; Hinze, H; Toscano, N. "Gingival Flap Attachment Healing with Amnion-Chorion Allograft Membrane: A Controlled, Split Mouth Case Report Replication of the Classic 1968 Hiatt Study." Journal of Implant & Advanced Clinical Dentistry. 2012;4(5):19-25.

Holtzclaw, D; Toscano, N. "Amnion-Chorion Allograft Barrier Used for Guided Tissue Regeneration Treatment of Periodontal Intrabony Defects: A Retrospective Observational Report." Clinical Advances in Periodontics. 2013;3(3):131-137.

Holtzclaw, D; Toscano, N. "BioXclude™ Placental Allograft Tissue Membrane Used in Combination with Bone Allograft for Site Preservation: A Case Series." Journal of Implant & Advanced Clinical Dentistry. 2011;3(3):35-50.

Hsu, GS. "Performing Transcanal Tympanoplasty with Human Amniotic Membrane Allograft." Otolaryngology – Head and Neck Surgery. 2013;149(2_suppl):234.

Hsu, GS. "Utilizing Dehydrated Human Amnion/Chorion Membrane Allograft in Transcanal Tympanoplasty." Otolaryngology. 2014;4(2):161.

Koob, TJ; Lim, JJ; Massee, M; Zabek, N; Denoziere, G. "Properties of Dehydrated Human Amnion/ Chorion Composite Grafts: Implications for Wound Repair and Soft Tissue Regeneration." Journal of Biomedical Materials Research – Part B: Applied Biomaterials. 2014;102(6):1353-1362.

Koob, TJ; Lim, JJ; Massee, M; Zabek, N; Rennert, R; Gurtner, G; Li, WW. "Angiogenic Properties of Dehydrated Human Amnion/Chorion Allografts: Therapeutic Potential for Soft Tissue Repair and Regeneration." Vascular Cell. 2014;6:10.

Koob, TJ; Lim, JJ; Zabek, N; Massee, M. "Cytokines in Single Layer Amnion Allografts Compared to Multilayer Amnion/Chorion Allografts for Wound Healing." Journal of Biomedical Materials Research – Part B: Applied Biomaterials. 2015;103(5):1133-1140.

Koob, TJ; Rennert, R: Zabek, N; Massee, M; Lim, JJ; Temenoff, JD; Li, WW; Gurtner, G. "Biological Properties of Dehydrated Human Amnion/Chorion Composite Graft: Implications for Chronic Wound Healing." International Wound Journal. 2013;10(5):493-500.

Lazzaro, D; Coe, R. "Repair of Limbal Dermoid With Excision and Placement of a Circumlimbal Pericardial Craft." Eye & Contact Lens. 2010;36(4):228-229.

Levin, B; Rubinstein, S; Rosenthaler, H; Fujiki, T; Tawil, P. "Advanced Surgical and Restorative Therapies Aimed at Rehabilitation of a Severe Dentoalveolar Defect in the Esthetic Zone." Journal of Implant & Advanced Clinical Dentistry. 2013;5(9): 17-27.

Li, W; Driver, V; Gould, L; Gibbons, G; Glat, P. "EpiFix Dehydrated Amnion/Chorion (dHACM) Therapy: The New Standard in Bioactive Wound Healing." Wounds. 2015;Supp:1-19.

Maan, ZN; Rennert, RC; Koob, TJ; Januszyk, M, Li, WW; Gurtner, GC. "Cell Recruitment by Amnion Chorion Grafts Promotes Neovascularization." Journal of Surgical Research. 2015;193(2):953-962.

Massee, M; Chinn, K; Lei, J; Lim, JJ; Young, CS; Koob, TJ. "Dehydrated Human Amnion/Chorion Membrane Regulates Stem Cell Activity In Vitro." Journal of Biomedical Materials Research – Part B: Applied Biomaterials. 2015;doi: 10.1002/jbm.b.33478.

Massee, M; Chinn, K; Lim, JJ; Godwin, L, Young, CS; Koob, TJ. "Type I and II Diabetic Adipose Derived Stem Cells Respond *In Vitro* to Dehydrated Human Amnion/Chorion Membrane Allograft Treatment by Increasing Proliferation, Migration, and Altering Cytokine Secretion." Advances in Wound Care. 2015;in press.

Mrugala, A; Sui, A; Plummer, M; Altman, I; Papineau, E; Frandsen, D; Hill, D; Ennis, WJ. "Amniotic Membrane Is a Potential Regenerative Option for Chronic Non-Healing Wounds: A Report of Five Cases Receiving Dehydrated Human Amnion/Chorion Membrane Allograft." International Wound Journal. 2015;DOI· 10.1111/iwj.12458.

Parekh, JG. "Surgical Pearls and Technique: Anterior Segment Ophthalmic Surgery." Advanced Ocular Care. 2012;May/June:22-23.

Parka, C: Kohanim; S; Zhu, L; Gehlbachb, P; and Chuck, R. "Immunosuppressive Property of Dried Human Amniotic Membrane." Ophthalmic Research. 2009;41:112-113.

Patel, VR; Samavedi, S; Bates, AS; Kumar, A; Coelho, Rocco, B; Palmer, K. "Dehydrated Human Amniotic Membrane Allograft Nerve Wrap Around the Prostatic Neurovascular Bundle Accelerates Early Return to Continence and Potency Following Robot-assisted Radical Prostatectomy: Propensity Score-matched Analysis." European Urology. 2015;67(6):977-980.

Penny, H; Rifkah, M; Weaver, A; Zaki, P; Young, A; Meloy, G; Flores, R. "Dehydrated Human Amnion/Chorion Tissue in Difficult-to-Heal DFUs: A Case Series." Journal of Wound Care. 2015;24(3):104-111.

Rosen, P. "Comprehensive Periodontal Regenerative Care: Combination Therapy Involving Bone Allograft, a Biologic, a Barrier, and a Subepithelial Connective Tissue Graft to Correct Hard- and Soft-Tissue Deformities." Clinical Advances in Periodontics. 2011;1(2):154-159.

148

Serena, TE; Carter, MJ; Le, LT; Sabo, MJ; DiMarco, DT; the EpiFix Study group. "A Multi-center Randomized Controlled Clinical Trial Evaluating the Use of Dehydrated Human Amnion/ Chorion Membrane Allografts and Multi-layer Compression Therapy vs. Multi-layer Compression Therapy Alone in the Treatment of Venous Leg Ulcers." Wound Repair and Regeneration. 2014;22(6):688-693.

Serena, TE; Carter, M; Le, L; Sabo, M; DiMarco, D. "Response to Letter from Dickerson and Slade." Wound Repair and Regeneration. 2015;23(1):143-144.

Shah, A. "Using Amniotic Membrane Allografts in the Treatment of Neuropathic Foot Ulcers." Journal of the American Podiatric Medical Association. 2014;104(2):198-202.

Sheikh, ES; Sheikh, ES; Fetterolf, DE. "Use of Dehydrated Human Amniotic Membrane Allografts to Promote Healing in Patients With Refractory Non Healing Wounds." International Wound Journal. 2014;11(6):711-717.

Subach, BR; Copay, AG. "The Use of a Dehydrated Amnion/Chorion Membrane Allograft in Patients Who Subsequently Undergo Re-exploration after Posterior Lumbar Instrumentation." Advances in Orthopedics. 2015;2015:Article ID 501202.

Tenenhaus, M; Greenberg, M; Potenza, B. "Dehydrated Human Amnion/Chorion Membrane for the Treatment of Severe Skin and Tissue Loss in an Preterm Infant: A Case Report." Journal of Wound Care. 2014;23(10):490-495.

Wallace, S. "Radiographic and Histomorphometric Analysis of Amniotic Allograft Tissue in Ridge Preservation: A Case Report." Journal of Implant & Advanced Clinical Dentistry. 2010;2(6):49-55.

Wallace, S; Cobb, C. "Histological and Computed Tomography Analysis of Amnion Chorion Membrane in Guided Bone Regeneration in Socket Augmentation." Journal of Implant & Advanced Clinical Dentistry. 2011;3(6):61-72.

Willett, NJ; Thote, T; Lin, AS; Moran, S; Raji, Y; Sridaran, S; Stevens, HY; Guldberg RE. "Intra-Articular Injection of Micronized Dehydrated Human Amnion/Chorion Membrane Attenuates Osteoarthritis Development." Arthritis Research and Therapy. 2014;16(1):R47.

Zelen, CM; Snyder, RJ; Serena, TE; Li, WW. "The Use of Human Amnion/Chorion Membrane in the Clinical Setting for Lower Extremity Repair: A Review." Clinics in Podiatric Medicine and Surgery. 2015;32(1):135-146.

Zelen, C. "An Evaluation of Dehydrated Human Amniotic Membrane Allografts in Patients with DFUs." Journal of Wound Care. 2013;22(7):347-348,350-351.

Zelen, C; Gould, L; Serena, T; Carter, M; Keller, J; Li, W. "A Prospective, Randomised, Controlled, Multi-Centre Comparative Effectiveness Study of Healing Using Dehydrated Human Amnion/ Chorion Membrane Allograft, Bioengineered Skin Substitute or Standard of Care for Treatment of Chronic Lower Extremity Diabetic Ulcers." International Wound Journal. 2014; DOI: 10.1111/ iwj.12395.

Zelen, C; Poka, A; Andrews, J. "Prospective, Randomized, Blinded, Comparative Study of Injectable Micronized Dehydrated Amniotic/Chorionic Membrane Allograft for Plantar Fasciitis A Feasibility Study." Foot and Ankle International. 2013;34(10):1332-1339.

Zelen, C; Serena, T; Fetterolf, D. "Dehydrated Human Amnion/Chorion Membrane Allografts in Patients with Chronic Diabetic Foot Ulcers: A Long-Term Follow-Up Study." Wound Medicine. 2014;4:1-4.

Zelen, C; Serena, T; Snyder, R. "A Prospective, Randomized Comparative Study of Weekly Versus Biweekly Application of Dehydrated Human Amnion/Chorion Membrane Allograft in the Management of Diabetic Foot Ulcers." International Wound Journal. 2014;11(2):122-128.

Zelen, C; Serena, T; Denoziere, G; and Fetterolf, D. "A Prospective Randomised Comparative Parallel Study of Amniotic Membrane Wound Graft in the Management of Diabetic Foot Ulcers." International Wound Journal. 2013;10(5): 502-507.

APPENDIX B: POSTER SESSION PRESENTATIONS ON MIMEDX dHACM ALLOGRAFTS

MiMedx Posters

Abrams, M. "Our Experience Utilizing Advanced Wound Therapy Combined with an Evidence-Based Approach to Threatening Wounds Reduces Amputations in the Caribbean Healthcare System." Desert Foot Conference. November 2012.

Abrebaya, A. "Efficacy of Particulate dHACM in Diabetic Foot Ulcerations, Chronic Lower Extremity Ulcerations and Other Wounds." Desert Foot Conference. November 2014.

Abrebaya, A. "AmnioFix Regenerative Injection in Achilles Tendinopathy." Desert Foot Conference. November 2013.

Allen, RT; Massie, J; Mahar, A; Phillips, F. "Preclinical Study of Human Allograft Amniotic Membrane as a Barrier to Epidural Fibrosis in the Early Wound of a Postlaminectomy Rat Model." International Society for the Advancement of Spine Surgery. April 2011.

Allen, RT; Massie, J; Mahar, A; Phillips, F. "Preclinical Study of Human Allograft Amniotic Membrane as a Barrier to Epidural Fibrosis in the Early Wound of a Postlaminectomy Rat Model." North American Spine Society. November 2011.

Bergquist, S. "Clinical and Cost Effectiveness of Dehydrated Human Amniotic/Chorionic Membrane Allografts for the Treatment of Non-Healing Wounds." Symposium on Advanced Wound Care. Fall 2013.

Bergquist, S. "Dehydrated Human Amnion/Chorion Membrane Allograft as a Treatment for Stage IV Pressure Ulcers." Symposium on Advanced Wound Care. September 2015.

Bergquist, S. "The Use of Dehydrated Human Amnion/Chorion Membrane for Treatment of Stage IV Pressure Ulcers." Symposium on Advanced Wound Care. October 2014.

Bergquist, S. "Treatment of Stage III and Stage IV Pressure Ulcers with Dehydrated Human Amnion/Chorion Membrane." Symposium on Advanced Wound Care. April 2014.

Bergquist, S. "Treatment of Stage III and Stage IV Pressure Ulcers with Dehydrated Human Amnion/Chorion Membrane." Wound Healing: Science & Industry Symposium. June 2014.

Bjorn, S; Kim, A. "Novel Approach to Expedite Chronic Wound Healing by Utilizing Injectable Dehydrated Amniotic Membrane." Desert Foot Conference. November 2012.

Bromley, C. "Dehydrated Human Amnion/Chorion Membrane Allograft for the Treatment of Chronic Ulceration in the Diabetic Patient." Desert Foot Conference. November 2014.

Chagares, W. "Healing Chronic Wounds Utilizing Dehydrated Human Amnion/Chorion Membrane (dHACM) Allografts Displaying Clinical and Cost Effectiveness in a Veteran and Department of Defense Population." Association of Military Surgeons of the United States. December 2014.

Chua, W. "Dehydrated Human Amnion/Chorion Membrane for the Treatment of Full-Thickness Plantar Burn in a Diabetic Patient: A Case Report." Desert Foot Conference. November 2013.

Chua, W. "Dehydrated Human Amnion/Chorion Membrane Particulate for the Treatment of Pressure Ulcers in Spinal Cord Injured Veterans: A Case Series of Three Healed Stage III Ulcers." Symposium on Advanced Wound Care. October 2014.

Chua, W. "Dehydrated Human Amniotic Membrane for the Treatment of Pressure Ulcers in Spinal Cord Injured Veterans: A Case Series." Symposium on Advanced Wound Care. Fall 2013.

Cole, W. "Pathologic Changes Observed with use of Micronized Dehydrated Human Amnion/Chorion Membrane Injections after Surgical Excision of Plantar Fibromatosis: a Unique Case Study." Symposium on Advanced Wound Care. September 2015.

Domass, M. "Healing Chronic Wounds Utilizing dHACM Allografts Displaying Clinical and Cost Effectiveness in A Veteran and DOD Population." Desert Foot Conference. November 2014.

Ennis, W; Sui, A; Papineau, E; Plummer M; Altman, I; Meneses, P. "Clinical Experience with a Novel Regenerative Template for Hard to Heal Wounds." Symposium on Advanced Wound Care. April 2012.

Farrer, D. "Dehisced Surgical Wound Secondary to Osteoectomy of Charcot Foot Treated with Purion® Processed Amniotic Tissue." Desert Foot Conference. November 2012.

Farrer, D. "Early Outcomes Utilizing PURION Processed Human Amniotic Membrane Allograft." Desert Foot Conference. November 2012.

Fetterolf, D; Istwan, N. "An Evaluation of Healing Metrics Associated with Commonly Used Advanced Wound Care Products for the Treatment of Chronic Diabetic Foot Ulcers." Symposium on Advanced Wound Care. October 2014.

Finkelstein, M. "Treatment of Refractory Wounds with Dehydrated Amniotic Membrane: A Case Series." Desert Foot Conference. November 2012.

Gaid, N; Tenenhaus, M; Greenberg, M; Potenza, B; Lee, J; Piatkowski, B. "Clinical Outcomes Following the Use of Dehydrated Human Amnion/Chorion Membrane in the Treatment of Severe Skin and Tissue Loss Resulting from Burn Injuries: A Case Series." Symposium on Advanced Wound Care. April 2015.

Garrett, M. "Clinical Experience with Dehydrated Human Amnion/Chorion Membrane Allografts for the Treatment of Chronic Foot and Leg Ulcers." Clinical Symposium on Advances in Skin & Wound Care. September-October 2014.

Giannikas, C; Udell, I; Steiner, A; Shih, C. "Sutureless Amniotic Membrane Transplantation for Ocular Surface Disorders: A Comparison of ProKera to AmbioDisc." Association for Research in Vision and Ophthalmology. May 2014.

Hansen, M; Anderson, J. "Chronic and Refractory Plantar Fasciitis Treatment with Single-Dose Dehydrated Amniotic Allograft Injection." American College of Foot and Ankle Surgeons. February 2013.

Harmon, L. "Experience with dHACM for a Complicated Sternal and Abdominal Wound." Desert Foot Conference. November 2013.

Harmon, LM. "Experience with dHACM for Chronic Lower Extremities Wounds and Pressure Ulcers." Desert Foot Conference. November 2014.

Hawkins, B. "Use of Dehydrated Human Amnion/Chorion Membrane Mesh Allograft in Wounds with Exposed Bone or Tendon." Symposium on Advanced Wound Care. September 2015.

Hawkins, B. "The Use of Particulate Dehydrated Human Amnion/Chorion Membrane Allograft for the Treatment of Diabetic Foot Ulcers." Symposium on Advanced Wound Care. April 2015.

Heath, L. "Application of Dehydrated Human Amnion/Chorion Membrane Allograft to Promote Healing of Recalcitrant Wounds in 16 Patients." Diabetic Limb Salvage. October 2014.

Heath, L. "Application of Dehydrated Human Amnion/Chorion Membrane Allograft to Promote Healing of Recalcitrant Wounds in 40 Patients." Desert Foot Conference. November 2014.

Hsu, G. "Performing Transcanal Tympanoplasty With Human Amniotic Membrane." American Academy of Ophthalmology. September-October 2013.

Jaffee, S; Tacktill, J; Mayo, D. "Dehydrated Human Amnion/Chorion Membrane Tissue Graft for the Treatment of Intractable Ulceration: A Series of Extraordinary Outliers." Symposium on Advanced Wound Care. Fall 2013.

Johnson R. "Clinical and Economic Impact of Utilizing Dehydrated Human Amnion/Chorion Membrane Allograft for the Treatment of Chronic Ulcers." American Podiatric Medical Association. July 2014.

Johnson, R. "Clinical and Economic Impact of Utilizing dHACM Allograft for the Treatment of Chronic Ulcers." Desert Foot Conference. November 2014.

Johnson, R. "Dehydrated Human Amnion/Chorion Membrane Allograft for the Treatment of a Post-Surgical Amputation Wound in a Diabetic Patient." American Podiatric Medical Association. July 2014.

Johnson, R. "Dehydrated Human Amnion/Chorion Membrane Allograft for the Treatment of a Post Surgical Amputation Wound in a Diabetic Patient." Desert Foot Conference. November 2013.

Kim, A. "New Technique to Deliver Micronized Dehydrated Amnion/Chorion Membrane Through Dermo-Jet Injection." Desert Foot Conference. November 2013.

Kim, A; Graves, D; Bjorn, S; Garoufalis, M. "Expediting Chronic Wound Healing by Utilizing Injectable Dehydrated Amniotic Membrane." American Podiatric Medical Association. July 2013.

Koob, T; Zabek, N; Massee, M; Waite, A. "Bioactive Properties of a Dehydrated Human Amniotic Membrane for Tissue Regeneration." Symposium on Advanced Wound Care. Fall 2012.

Lenz, R; Park, H; Nagesh, D. "Dehydrated Human Amnion/Chorion Membrane in Conjunction with Total Contact Cast for Treatment of Plantar Diabetic Foot Ulceration." Desert Foot Conference. November 2014.

Lorne, K; Varca, P. "Retrospective Case study of a Chronic Neuropathic Wound Healed with dHACM Allografts in the VA Setting." Desert Foot Conference. November 2014.

Massee, M; Chinn, K; Lei, J; Lim, JJ; Young, CS; Koob, TJ. "Dehydrated Human Amnion/Chorion Membrane Regulates Stem Cell Activity In Vitro." Symposium on Advanced Wound Care. September 2015.

Massee, M; Chinn, K; Lim, JJ; Godwin, L, Young, CS; Koob, TJ. "Type I and II Diabetic Adipose Derived Stem Cells Respond In Vitro to Dehydrated Human Amnion/Chorion Membrane Allograft Treatment by Increasing Proliferation, Migration, and Altering Cytokine Secretion." Symposium on Advanced Wound Care. September 2015.

Nagesh, D; Lenz, R; Park, H; Sanchez, P; Ruff, J; Garoufalis, M. "The Use of Dehydrated Human Amnion/Chorion Membrane (dHACM) Allografts to Expedite Healing in Patients with Five Major Types of Refractory Non-Healing Wounds: A Cohort Study." Desert Foot Conference. November 2014.

O'Donnell, E. "EpiFix – Human Amniotic Membrane Allograft Use in the Treatment of Chronic Diabetic Wounds." Clinical Symposium on Advances in Skin and Wound Care. September-October 2010.

Pantera, P. "Application of Amniotic Tissue Has Accelerated Healing of Plantar Hallux Ulcer." Desert Foot Conference. November 2012.

Park, H. "Hypergranular Wounds Secondary to Surgical Dehiscence Treated with Dehydrated Human Amnion/Chorion." Desert Foot Conference. November 2014.

Pichika, R; Le, Y; Yamaguchi, T; Garfin, S; Drapeau, S; Fujiwara, T; Lenz, M; Sakai, D; Masuda, K. "Suppressive Effect of Injectable Micronized Amniotic Membrane Particles on Inflammatory Cytokines In Vitro Human Intervertebral Disc Explant Cultures." Orthopaedic Research Society and International Society for the Advancement of Spine Surgery. 2014.

Pougatsch. "Human Amniotic Membrane Allograft to Treat Diabetic Foot Ulcers with Exposed Bone and Tendon." Symposium on Advanced Wound Care. April 2014.

Rifleman, G. "The Use of Dehydrated Human Amnion/Chorion Membrane to Treat a Large Dorsal Wound With Exposed Tendons and Deep Tracking: A Retrospective Case Study Review of One Patient in a VA Setting." Minneapolis VA Hospital. June 2015.

Sanchez, P. "An Innovative Dehydrated Human Amnion/Chorion Membrane (dHACM) Application Technique for Large VLUs: A Case Study." American Podiatric Medical Association. July 2015.

Sanchez, P; Lenz, RC; Nagesh, D; Park, H; Ruff, J; Park, S; Garoufalis, M. "An Innovative dHACM Membrane Application Technique for Large VLUs: A Case study." Desert Foot Conference. November 2014.

Sears, A; Meredith, A; Patterson, B; Cikrit, D; Roudebush, R. "Treatment of Lower Extremity Chronic Wounds with Dehydrated Human Amnion/Chorion Membrane (dHACM): A Vascular Compromised Cohort (ABI<.65)." Desert Foot Conference. November 2013.

Serena; TE; Fetterolf, D; Harris, S; Doner, B; Patel, K; Sabo, M; Demarco, D; Lullove, E; Le, L; Shettel, C; McConnell, S; Connell, H. "A Multi-center Randomized Controlled Clinical Trial of Dehydrated Human Amnion/Chorion Membrane and Standard of Care vs. Standard of Care Alone in the Treatment of Venous Leg Ulcers." Symposium on Advanced Wound Care. April 2014.

Serena, T; Carter, M; EpiFix VLU Study group. "Does Application of Dehydrated Human Amnion/ Chorion Membrane (dHACM) Increase Matrix Metalloproteinase Levels in Wounds?" Symposium on Advanced Wound Care. September 2015.

Serena, T; Fetterolf, D. "Clinical Research: Dehydrated Human Amniotic Membrane (dHAM) Treatment of Lower Extremity Venous Ulceration." Symposium on Advanced Wound Care. April 2012.

Serena, T; Yaakov, R; DiMarco, D; Le, L; Taffe, E; Donaldson, M; Miller, M. "Evaluation of a Surrogate Outcome Used in a Study of Dehydrated Human Amnion/Chorion Membrane for the Treatment of Venous Leg Ulcers." Symposium on Advanced Wound Care. April 2015.

Shah, A. "Human Amniotic Membrane Allograft for Treatment in Diabetic Wound Care Management." Diabetic Wound Care Management PMA. July 2011.

Shah, A. "Human Amniotic Membrane Allograft for Treatment in Diabetic Wound Care Management." Advances in Skin and Wound Care. September-October 2010.

Shah, N; Catanzano, A; Chahine, N; Razzano,P; Grande, D. "Evaluation of Achilles Tendon Repair Enhanced with Amniotic Membrane-derived Allografts." Orthopaedic Research Society. January 2011.

Sheikh, E. "Use of Dehydrated Human Amniotic Membrane (dHAM) Allografts to Promote Healing in Patients with Refractory Non-Healing Wounds." Symposium on Advanced Wound Care. Fall 2013.

Sheikh, E. "Use of Dehydrated Human Amniotic Membrane (dHAM) Allografts to Promote Healing in Patients with Refractory Non-Healing Wounds." Symposium on Advanced Wound Care. Spring 2013.

Snyder, R. "Dehydrated Human Amnion/Chorion Membrane as Adjunctive Therapy in the Treatment of Pyoderma Gangrenosum: A Case Report." Symposium on Advanced Wound Care. September 2015.

Stuck, R. "Injectable PURION Processed Dehydrated Amniotic Membrane Use in Patient with Rupture of the Plantar Fascia." Desert Foot Conference. November 2012.

Taddie, KL. "A Retrospective View of the Treatment of Chronic Lower Extremity Wounds with dHACM." Desert Foot Conference. November 2014.

Talis, R; Ahrens, A. "Description of Technique for Implantation of Dehydrated Human Amnion/ Chorion Membrane Allograft for the Treatment of Plantar Fasciitis." Symposium on Advanced Wound Care. Sept 2015.

Tenenhaus, M; Gaid, N. "Dehydrated Human Amnion/Chorion Membrane for the Treatment of Severe Skin and Tissue Loss Resulting from Congenital Candidiasis in an Extremely Preterm Infant: A Unique Case Report." Symposium on Advanced Wound Care. October 2014.

Terebessy, J. "Retrospective Analysis of Chronic Wounds Healed with dHACM Allografts in the VA Setting." Desert Foot Conference. November 2014.

Serena, T; Istwan, N; Stanziano, G; Fetterolf, D. "Clinical Factors and Cost Effectiveness Associated with Healing of Venous Leg Ulcers with Dehydrated Human Amnion/Chorion Membrane Allografts." Symposium on Advanced Wound Care. September 2015.

Warner, J; Warner, K. "Use of Dehydrated Human Amnion Chorion Membrane Allograft for Reconstruction of Mohs Micrographic Surgical Defects and Dehisced Wounds." American College of Mohs Surgeons. May 2013.

Weinman, J; Broner, T. "Dehydrated Human Amnion/Chorion Membrane (dHACM) Injectable for Lower Extremity Tendinopathies." Desert Foot Conference. November 2014.

Weiszbicki, B. "Our Experience with an Evidenced Based Approach to treating Diabetic Foot Ulcers (DFU) for the Prevention of Amputations in Veterans Everywhere (PAVE) using Advanced Therapies." Desert Foot Conference. November 2012.

Werkhoven, G. "The Use of Epifix Allograft Implication to Treat Chronic Diabetic Foot Ulcers IN Refractory and Non-Refractory Patients: A Retrospective Case Study Review of Five Patients in a VA Setting." Desert Foot Conference. November 2012.

Willett, N; Lin, A; Thote, T; Raji, Y; Moran, S: Stevens, H; Guldberg, R. "Micronized Amnion Attenuates Osteoarthritis Disease Progression in a Rat Model." Hilton Head Regenerative Medicine Symposium. March 2012.

Xenoudi, P; Lucas, M. "Comparison of Porcine and Amnion Chorion Resorbable Collagen Membranes using Immunohistochemistry." International Association of Dental Research. March 2011.

Xiong, K. "EpiFix Utilization for Advanced Wound Therapy in an Evidence Based Approach to Treat Foot Ulcers." Desert Foot Conference. November 2013.

Zelen, C. "A Long-term Follow-up Study of Chronic Diabetic Foot Ulcers Healed with Dehydrated Human Amniotic/Chorionic Membrane Allografts". Clinical Symposium on Advances in Skin and Wound Care. October 2013.

Zelen, C. "A Prospective, Randomised, Controlled, Multi-Centre Comparative Effectiveness Study of Healing Using Dehydrated Human Amnion/Chorion Membrane Allograft, Bioengineered Skin Substitute, or Standard of Care for Treatment of Chronic Diabetic Lower Extremity Ulcers." American Podiatric Medical Association. July 2015.

Zelen, C. "An Evaluation of Healing with the use of Dehydrated Human Amniotic/Chorionic Membrane Allografts following Failure of Standard of Care in Patients with Chronic Diabetic Foot Ulcers." American Podiatric Medical Association. July 2013.

Zelen, C; Poka, A; Andrews, J. "A Prospective, Randomized, Blinded, Comparative Study of Injectable Dehydrated Human Amniotic/Chorionic Membrane (dHACM) in the Treatment of Recalcitrant Plantar Fasciitis." American Orthopaedic Foot and Ankle Society. July 2013.

Zelen, C; Serena, T. "Human Amniotic Membrane in the Treatment of Non-Healing Diabetic Foot Ulcers: A Prospective Randomized Controlled Trial." Symposium on Advanced Wound Care. May 2013.

Zelen, C; Serena, T; Fetterolf, D. "A Long-term Follow-up Study of Chronic Diabetic Foot Ulcers Healed with Dehydrated Human Amniotic/Chorionic Membrane Allografts." Symposium on Advanced Wound Care. Fall 2013.

Zelen, C; Serena, T; Fetterolf, D. "Human Amniotic Membrane in the Treatment of Non-Healing Diabetic Foot Ulcers: A Randomized Controlled Trial." Clinical Symposium on Advances in Skin and Wound Care. October 2012.

Zelen, C; Serena, T; Fetterolf, D. "Recurrence of Chronic Diabetic Foot Ulcers Healed with Dehydrated Human Amnion/Chorion Membrane Allografts: A Long-term Follow-up Study." American Professional Wound Care Association. March 2014.

Zelen, C; Serena, T; Gould, L: Keller, J; Carter, M; Li, W "A Prospective, Randomized, Controlled, Multi-Center Comparative Effectiveness Study of Healing Using Dehydrated Human Amnion/ Chorion Membrane Allograft, Bioengineered Skin Substitute, or Standard of Care for Treatment of Chronic Diabetic Lower Extremity Ulcers." Symposium on Advanced Wound Care. April 2015.

Zelen, C; Serena, T; Gould, L; Lang, A; Keller, J; Carter, M; Li, W. "A Prospective, Randomized, Controlled, Multi-Center Comparative Effectiveness Study of Healing Using Dehydrated Human Amnion/Chorion Membrane Allograft, Bioengineered Skin Substitute, or Standard of Care for Treatment of Chronic Diabetic Lower Extremity Ulcers." American College of Foot and Ankle Surgeons. February 2015.

Zelen, C; Serena, T; Snyder, R. "A Prospective, Randomized Comparative Study of Weekly versus Biweekly Application of Dehydrated Human Amnion/Chorion Membrane Allograft in the Management of Diabetic Foot Ulcers." American Podiatric Medical Association. July 2014.

Zelen, C; Serena, T; Snyder, R. "A Prospective, Randomized Comparative Study of Weekly versus Biweekly Application of Dehydrated Human Amnion/Chorion Membrane Allograft in the Management of Diabetic Foot Ulcers." American Professional Wound Care Association. March 2014.

Zelen, C; Serena, T; Snyder, R. "A Prospective, Randomized Comparative Study of Weekly versus Biweekly Application of Dehydrated Human Amnion/Chorion Membrane Allograft in the Management of Diabetic Foot Ulcers." Symposium on Advanced Wound Care. April 2014.

Zelen, C; Tackhill, J; Serena, T. "A Long-term Follow-up Study of Chronic Diabetic Foot Ulcers Healed with Dehydrated Human Amnion/Chorion Membrane Allografts." American College of Foot and Ankle Surgeons. February-March 2014.

Zhu, L. "Immunosuppressive Property of Dried Human Amniotic Membrane." Association for Research in Vision and Ophthalmology. May 2007.

REFERENCES

1. Martin, P. and S.J. Leibovich, *Inflammatory cells during wound repair: the good, the bad and the ugly.* Trends Cell Biol, 2005. 15(11): p. 599-607.

2. Park, J.E. and A. Barbul, *Understanding the role of immune regulation in wound healing.* Am J Surg, 2004. 187(5A): p. 11S-16S.

3. Cassatella, M.A., *Neutrophil-derived proteins: selling cytokines by the pound.* Adv Immunol, 1999. 73: p. 369-509.

4. Artuc, M., B. Hermes, U.M. Steckelings, et al., *Mast cells and their mediators in cutaneous wound healing-- active participants or innocent bystanders?* Exp Dermatol, 1999. 8(1): p. 1-16.

5. Iba, Y., A. Shibata, M. Kato, et al., *Possible involvement of mast cells in collagen remodeling in the late phase of cutaneous wound healing in mice.* Int Immunopharmacol, 2004. 4(14): p. 1873-80.

6. Gregorio, J., S. Meller, C. Conrad, et al., *Plasmacytoid dendritic cells sense skin injury and promote wound healing through type I interferons.* J Exp Med, 2010. 207(13): p. 2921-30.

7. Gillitzer, R. and M. Goebeler, *Chemokines in cutaneous wound healing.* J Leukoc Biol, 2001. 69(4): p. 513-21.

8. Duffield, J.S., *The inflammatory macrophage: a story of Jekyll and Hyde.* Clin Sci (Lond), 2003. 104(1): p. 27-38.

9. Gordon, S., *Alternative activation of macrophages.* Nat Rev Immunol, 2003. 3(1): p. 23-35.

10. Ma, J., T. Chen, J. Mandelin, et al., *Regulation of macrophage activation.* Cell Mol Life Sci, 2003. 60(11): p. 2334-46.

11. Huang, S., W. Hendriks, A. Althage, et al., *Immune response in mice that lack the interferon-gamma receptor.* Science, 1993. 259(5102): p. 1742-5.

12. Janeway, C.A., Jr. and R. Medzhitov, *Innate immune recognition.* Annu Rev Immunol, 2002. 20: p. 197-216.

13. Luster, A.D., *The role of chemokines in linking innate and adaptive immunity.* Curr Opin Immunol, 2002. 14(1): p. 129-35.

14. Chizzolini, C., R. Rezzonico, C. De Luca, et al., *Th2 cell membrane factors in association with IL-4 enhance matrix metalloproteinase-1 (MMP-1) while decreasing MMP-9 production by granulocyte-macrophage colony-stimulating factor-differentiated human monocytes.* J Immunol, 2000. 164(11): p. 5952-60.

15. Gibbs, D.F., R.L. Warner, S.J. Weiss, et al., *Characterization of matrix metalloproteinases produced by rat alveolar macrophages.* Am J Respir Cell Mol Biol, 1999. 20(6): p. 1136-44.

16. Stein, M., S. Keshav, N. Harris, et al., *Interleukin 4 potently enhances murine macrophage mannose receptor activity: a marker of alternative immunologic macrophage activation.* J Exp Med, 1992. 176(1): p. 287-92.

17. Doherty, T.M., R. Kastelein, S. Menon, et al., *Modulation of murine macrophage function by IL-13.* J Immunol, 1993. 151(12): p. 7151-60.

18. Andrew, D.P., M.S. Chang, J. McNinch, et al., *STCP-1 (MDC) CC chemokine acts specifically on chronically activated Th2 lymphocytes and is produced by monocytes on stimulation with Th2 cytokines IL-4 and IL-13.* J Immunol, 1998. 161(9): p. 5027-38.

19. Imai, T., M. Nagira, S. Takagi, et al., *Selective recruitment of CCR4-bearing Th2 cells toward antigen-presenting cells by the CC chemokines thymus and activation-regulated chemokine and macrophage-derived chemokine.* Int Immunol, 1999. 11(1): p. 81-8.

20. Kodelja, V., C. Muller, O. Politz, et al., *Alternative macrophage activation-associated CC-chemokine-1, a novel structural homologue of macrophage inflammatory protein-1 alpha with a Th2-associated expression pattern.* J Immunol, 1998. 160(3): p. 1411-8.

21. Goerdt, S., O. Politz, K. Schledzewski, et al., *Alternative versus classical activation of macrophages.* Pathobiology, 1999. 67(5-6): p. 222-6.

22. Mantovani, A., M. Locati, A. Vecchi, et al., *Decoy receptors: a strategy to regulate inflammatory cytokines and chemokines.* Trends Immunol, 2001. 22(6): p. 328-36.

23. Mosser, D.M., *The many faces of macrophage activation.* J Leukoc Biol, 2003. 73(2): p. 209-12.

24. Song, E., N. Ouyang, M. Horbelt, et al., *Influence of alternatively and classically activated macrophages on fibrogenic activities of human fibroblasts.* Cell Immunol, 2000. 204(1): p. 19-28.

25. Sunderkotter, C., M. Goebeler, K. Schulze-Osthoff, et al., *Macrophage-derived angiogenesis factors.* Pharmacol Ther, 1991. 51(2): p. 195-216.

26. Hesse, M., M. Modolell, A.C. La Flamme, et al., *Differential regulation of nitric oxide synthase-2 and arginase-1 by type 1/type 2 cytokines in vivo: granulomatous pathology is shaped by the pattern of L-arginine metabolism.* J Immunol, 2001. 167(11): p. 6533-44.

27. Munder, M., K. Eichmann, and M. Modolell, *Alternative metabolic states in murine macrophages reflected by the nitric oxide synthase/arginase balance: competitive regulation by CD4+ T cells correlates with Th1/Th2 phenotype.* J Immunol, 1998. 160(11): p. 5347-54.

28. Morris, S.M., Jr., D. Kepka-Lenhart, and L.C. Chen, *Differential regulation of arginases and inducible nitric oxide synthase in murine macrophage cells.* Am J Physiol, 1998. 275(5 Pt 1): p. E740-7.

29. Koh, T.J. and L.A. DiPietro, *Inflammation and wound healing: the role of the macrophage.* Expert Rev Mol Med, 2011. 13: p. e23.

30. Barbul, A., R.J. Breslin, J.P. Woodyard, et al., *The effect of in vivo T helper and T suppressor lymphocyte depletion on wound healing.* Ann Surg, 1989. 209(4): p. 479-83.

31. Wilgus, T.A., *Immune cells in the healing skin wound: influential players at each stage of repair.* Pharmacol Res, 2008. 58(2): p. 112-6.

32. Singer, A.J. and R.A. Clark, *Cutaneous wound healing.* N Engl J Med, 1999. 341(10): p. 738-46.

33. Tonnesen, M.G., X. Feng, and R.A. Clark, *Angiogenesis in wound healing.* J Investig Dermatol Symp Proc, 2000. 5(1): p. 40-6.

34. Loffek, S., O. Schilling, and C.W. Franzke, *Biological role of matrix metalloproteinases: a critical balance.* Eur Respir J, 2011. 38(1): p. 191-208.

35. Lu, P., K. Takai, V.M. Weaver, et al., *Extracellular matrix degradation and remodeling in development and disease.* Cold Spring Harb Perspect Biol, 2011. 3(12).

36. Stadelmann, W.K., A.G. Digenis, and G.R. Tobin, *Physiology and healing dynamics of chronic cutaneous wounds.* Am J Surg, 1998. 176(2A Suppl): p. 26S-38S.

37. Shaw, T.J. and P. Martin, *Wound repair at a glance.* J Cell Sci, 2009. 122(Pt 18): p. 3209-13.

38. Serena, T., B. Cullen, S. Bayliff, et al. *Protease Activity Levels Associated with Healing Status of Chronic Wounds.* 2011; Available from: http://www.systagenix.com/cms/uploads/NG42-11-final-Serena-et-al-Protease-Activity-Levels-Associated-with-Healing-Status-of-Chronic-Wounds-Serena-Group-et-al.pdf.

39. Menke, N.B., K.R. Ward, T.M. Witten, et al., *Impaired wound healing.* Clin Dermatol, 2007. 25(1): p. 19-25.

40. Norbury, K.C. and M.P. Moyer, *Effect of negative pressure therapy on the inflammatory response of the intestinal microenvironment in a porcine septic model.* Mediators Inflamm, 2015. DOI: 10.1155/2015/419841.

41. Wu, K.H., X.M. Mo, Z.C. Han, et al., *Stem cell engraftment and survival in the ischemic heart.* Ann Thorac Surg, 2011. 92(5): p. 1917-25.

42. Hocking, A.M. and N.S. Gibran, *Mesenchymal stem cells: paracrine signaling and differentiation during cutaneous wound repair.* Exp Cell Res, 2010. 316(14): p. 2213-9.

43. Volarevic, V., N. Arsenijevic, M.L. Lukic, et al., *Concise review: Mesenchymal stem cell treatment of the complications of diabetes mellitus.* Stem Cells, 2011. 29(1): p. 5-10.

44. Griffiths, M., N. Ojeh, R. Livingstone, et al., *Survival of Apligraf in acute human wounds.* Tissue Eng, 2004. 10(7-8): p. 1180-95.

45. Hu, S., R.S. Kirsner, V. Falanga, et al., *Evaluation of Apligraf persistence and basement membrane restoration in donor site wounds: a pilot study.* Wound Repair Regen, 2006. 14(4): p. 427-33.

46. Jones, I., L. Currie, and R. Martin, *A guide to biological skin substitutes.* Br J Plast Surg, 2002. 55(3): p. 185-93.

47. Zelen, C.M., L. Gould, T.E. Serena, et al., *A prospective, randomised, controlled, multi-centre comparative effectiveness study of healing using dehydrated human amnion/chorion membrane allograft, bioengineered skin substitute or standard of care for treatment of chronic lower extremity diabetic ulcers.* Int Wound J, 2014.

48. Wainwright, D.J., *Use of an acellular allograft dermal matrix (AlloDerm) in the management of full-thickness burns.* Burns, 1995. 21(4): p. 243-8.

49. Weiland, A.J., T.W. Phillips, and M.A. Randolph, *Bone grafts: a radiologic, histologic, and biomechanical model comparing autografts, allografts, and free vascularized bone grafts.* Plast Reconstr Surg, 1984. 74(3): p. 368-79.

50. Peterson, R.K., W.R. Shelton, and A.L. Bomboy, *Allograft versus autograft patellar tendon anterior cruciate ligament reconstruction: A 5-year follow-up.* Arthroscopy, 2001. 17(1): p. 9-13.

51. Chiu, T. and A. Burd, *"Xenograft" dressing in the treatment of burns.* Clin Dermatol, 2005. 23(4): p. 419-23.

52.   Badylak, S., K. Kokini, B. Tullius, et al., *Morphologic study of small intestinal submucosa as a body wall repair device.* J Surg Res, 2002. 103(2): p. 190-202.

53.   Freytes, D.O., R.S. Tullius, J.E. Valentin, et al., *Hydrated versus lyophilized forms of porcine extracellular matrix derived from the urinary bladder.* J Biomed Mater Res A, 2008. 87(4): p. 862-72.

54.   Daniel, J., R. Tofe, R. Spencer, et al., inventors; MiMedx Group, Inc (Kennesaw, GA), assignee. *Placental tissue grafts* 2012. U.S. Patent 8,323,701.

55.   Daniel, J., R. Tofe, R. Spencer, et al., inventors; MiMedx Group, Inc (Kennesaw, GA), assignee. *Placental tissue grafts.* 2013. U.S. Patent 8,357,403.

56.   Daniel, J., inventor; MiMedx Group, Inc (Kennesaw, GA), assignee. *Placental tissue grafts.* 2013. U.S. Patent 8,372,437.

57.   Daniel, J., R. Tofe, R. Spencer, et al., inventors; MiMedx Group, Inc (Kennesaw, GA), assignee. *Method for inhibiting adhesion formation using an improved placental tissue graft.* 2013. U.S. Patent 8,372,438.

58.   Daniel, J., R. Tofe, R. Spencer, et al., inventors; MiMedx Group, Inc (Kennesaw, GA), assignee. *Method for treating a wound using improved placental tissue graft.* 2013. U.S. Patent 8,372,439.

59.   Daniel, J., R. Tofe, R. Spencer, et al., inventors; MiMedx Group, Inc (Kennesaw, GA), assignee. *Placental tissue grafts.* 2012. U.S. Patent 8,409,626.

60.   Daniel, J., inventor; MiMedx Group, Inc (Kennesaw, GA), assignee. *Placental tissue grafts.* 2013. U.S. Patent 8,460,715.

61.   Daniel, J., inventor; MiMedx Group, Inc (Kennesaw, GA), assignee. *Method for applying a label to a placental tissue graft.* 2013. U.S. Patent 8,460,716.

62.   Daniel, J., inventor; MiMedx Group, Inc (Kennesaw, GA), assignee. *Methods for determining the orientation of a tissue graft.* 2013. U.S. Patent 8,597,687.

63.   Daniel, J., inventor; MiMedx Group, Inc (Kennesaw, GA), assignee. *Placental graft.* 2014. U.S. Patent 8,623,421.

64.   Daniel, J., R. Spencer, J. Russo, et al., inventors; MiMedx Group, Inc (Kennesaw, GA), assignee. *Placental tissue grafts.* 2014. U.S. Patent 8,642,092.

65.   Daniel, J., R. Tofe, R. Spencer, et al., inventors; MiMedx Group, Inc (Kennesaw, GA), assignee. *Placental tissue grafts.* 2014. U.S. Patent 8,703,206.

66.   Daniel, J., R. Spencer, J. Russo, et al., inventors; MiMedx Group, Inc (Kennesaw, GA), assignee. *Placental tissue grafts.* 2014. U.S. Patent 8,703,207.

67.   Daniel, J., R. Tofe, R. Spencer, et al., inventors; MiMedx Group, Inc (Kennesaw, GA), assignee. *Placental tissue grafts.* 2014. U.S. Patent 8,709,493.

68.   Daniel, J., inventor; MiMedx Group, Inc (Marietta, GA), assignee. *Placental tissue grafts.* 2014. U.S. Patent 8,709,494.

69.   Pringle, D. and M. Lepeak, inventors; MiMedx Group, Inc (Marietta, GA), assignee. *Dehydration device and methods for drying biological materials.* 2014. U.S. Patent 8,904,664.

70.   Daniel, J., R. Tofe, R. Spencer, et al., inventors; MiMedx Group, Inc (Marietta, GA), assignee. *Placental tissue grafts.* 2015. U.S. Patent 8,932,643.

71.   Ramakrishnan, K.M. and V. Jayaraman, *Management of partial-thickness burn wounds by amniotic membrane: a cost-effective treatment in developing countries.* Burns, 1997. 23 Suppl 1: p. S33-6.

72.   Niknejad, H., H. Peirovi, M. Jorjani, et al., *Properties of the amniotic membrane for potential use in tissue engineering.* Eur Cell Mater, 2008. 15: p. 88-99.

73.   Koob, T.J., R. Rennert, N. Zabek, et al., *Biological properties of dehydrated human amnion/chorion composite graft: implications for chronic wound healing.* Int Wound J, 2013. 10(5): p. 493-500.

74.   Koob, T.J., J.J. Lim, M. Massee, et al., *Properties of dehydrated human amnion/chorion composite grafts: Implications for wound repair and soft tissue regeneration.* J Biomed Mater Res B Appl Biomater, 2014. 102(6): p. 1353-62.

75.   Koob, T.J., J.J. Lim, M. Massee, et al., *Angiogenic properties of dehydrated human amnion/chorion allografts: therapeutic potential for soft tissue repair and regeneration.* Vasc Cell, 2014. 6: p. 10.

76.   Koob, T.J., J.J. Lim, N. Zabek, et al., *Cytokines in single layer amnion allografts compared to multilayer amnion/chorion allografts for wound healing.* J Biomed Mater Res B Appl Biomater, 2015. 103(5): p. 1133-40.

77.   Maan, Z.N., R.C. Rennert, T.J. Koob, et al., *Cell recruitment by amnion chorion grafts promotes neovascularization.* J Surg Res, 2015. 193(2): p. 953-62.

78. Massee, M., K. Chinn, J. Lei, et al., *Dehydrated human amnion/chorion membrane regulates stem cell activity in vitro*. J Biomed Mater Res B Appl Biomater, 2015. DOI: 10.1002/jbm.b.33478.

79. Massee, M., K. Chinn, J.J. Lim, et al., *Type I and II diabetic adipose derived stem cells respond in vitro to dehydrated human amnion/chorion membrane allograft treatment by increasing proliferation, migration, and altering cytokine secretion*. Adv Wound Care, 2015. in press.

80. Zelen, C.M., T.E. Serena, G. Denoziere, et al., *A prospective randomised comparative parallel study of amniotic membrane wound graft in the management of diabetic foot ulcers*. Int Wound J, 2013. 10(5): p. 502-7.

81. Zelen, C.M., T.E. Serena, and D.E. Fetterolf, *Dehydrated human amnion/chorion membrane allografts in patients with chronic diabetic foot ulcers: A long-term follow-up study*. Wound Medicine, 2014. 4: p. 1-4.

82. Zelen, C.M., A. Poka, and J. Andrews, *Prospective, randomized, blinded, comparative study of injectable micronized dehydrated amniotic/chorionic membrane allograft for plantar fasciitis--a feasibility study*. Foot Ankle Int, 2013. 34(10): p. 1332-9.

83. Zelen, C.M., *An evaluation of dehydrated human amniotic membrane allografts in patients with DFUs*. J Wound Care, 2013. 22(7): p. 347-8, 350-1.

84. Zelen, C.M., T.E. Serena, and R.J. Snyder, *A prospective, randomised comparative study of weekly versus biweekly application of dehydrated human amnion/chorion membrane allograft in the management of diabetic foot ulcers*. Int Wound J, 2014. 11(2): p. 122-8.

85. Sheikh, E.S., E.S. Sheikh, and D.E. Fetterolf, *Use of dehydrated human amniotic membrane allografts to promote healing in patients with refractory non healing wounds*. Int Wound J, 2014. 11(6): p. 711-7.

86. Forbes, J. and D.E. Fetterolf, *Dehydrated amniotic membrane allografts for the treatment of chronic wounds: a case series*. J Wound Care, 2012. 21(6): p. 290, 292, 294-6.

87. Fetterolf, D.E. and R. Savage, *Dehydrated human amniotic tissue improves healing time, cost of care*. Today's Wound Clinic, 2013. January/February: p. 19-20.

88. Fetterolf, D.E. and R.J. Snyder, *Scientific and Clinical Support for the Use of Dehydrated Amniotic Membrane in Wound Management*. Wounds, 2012. 24(10): p. 299-307.

89. Shah, A.P., *Using amniotic membrane allografts in the treatment of neuropathic foot ulcers*. J Am Podiatr Med Assoc, 2014. 104(2): p. 198-202.

90. Hsu, G.S., *Utilizing Dehydrated Human Amnion/Chorion Membrane Allograft in Transcanal Tympanoplasty*. Otolaryngology, 2014. 4(2): p. 161.

91. Willett, N.J., T. Thote, A.S. Lin, et al., *Intra-articular injection of micronized dehydrated human amnion/chorion membrane attenuates osteoarthritis development*. Arthritis Res Ther, 2014. 16(1): p. R47.

92. Fetterolf, D.E., N.B. Istwan, and G.J. Stanziano, *An Evaluation of Healing Metrics Associated With Commonly Used Advanced Wound Care Products For the Treatment of Chronic Diabetic Foot Ulcers*. Managed Care, 2014. July: p. 31-38.

93. Serena, T.E., M.J. Carter, L.T. Le, et al., *A multicenter, randomized, controlled clinical trial evaluating the use of dehydrated human amnion/chorion membrane allografts and multilayer compression therapy vs. multilayer compression therapy alone in the treatment of venous leg ulcers*. Wound Repair Regen, 2014. 22(6): p. 688-93.

94. Subach, B.R. and A.G. Copay, *The use of a dehydrated amnion/chorion membrane allograft in patients who subsequently undergo reexploration after posterior lumbar instrumentation*. Adv Orthop, 2015. 2015: p. 501202.

95. Dua, H.S., J.A. Gomes, A.J. King, et al., *The amniotic membrane in ophthalmology*. Surv Ophthalmol, 2004. 49(1): p. 51-77.

96. Gude, N.M., C.T. Roberts, B. Kalionis, et al., *Growth and function of the normal human placenta*. Thromb Res, 2004. 114(5-6): p. 397-407.

97. Parry, S. and J.F. Strauss, *Premature rupture of the fetal membranes*. N Engl J Med, 1998. 338(10): p. 663-70.

98. Oyen, M.L., R.F. Cook, and S.E. Calvin, *Mechanical failure of human fetal membrane tissues*. J Mater Sci Mater Med, 2004. 15(6): p. 651-8.

99. Chua, W.K. and M.L. Oyen, *Do we know the strength of the chorioamnion? A critical review and analysis*. Eur J Obstet Gynecol Reprod Biol, 2009. 144 Suppl 1: p. S128-33.

100. Bourne, G., *The foetal membranes. A review of the anatomy of normal amnion and chorion and some aspects of their function*. Postgrad Med J, 1962. 38: p. 193-201.

101. Lee, J.S., R. Romero, Y.M. Han, et al., *Placenta-on-a-chip: a novel platform to study the biology of the human placenta*. J Matern Fetal Neonatal Med, 2015: p. 1-9.

159

102. Sobolewski, K., E. Bankowski, L. Chyczewski, et al., *Collagen and glycosaminoglycans of Wharton's jelly.* Biol Neonate, 1997. 71(1): p. 11-21.

103. Underwood, M.A., W.M. Gilbert, and M.P. Sherman, *Amniotic fluid: not just fetal urine anymore.* J Perinatol, 2005. 25(5): p. 341-8.

104. Koob, T.J., J.J. Lim, N. Zabek, et al., *Cytokines in single layer amnion allografts compared to multilayer amnion/chorion allografts for wound healing.* J Biomed Mater Res B Appl Biomater, 2014. DOI: 10.1002/jbm.b.33265.

105. MiMedx Research Report. MM-RD-00001: Evaluation of Growth Factors in EpiFix, AmnioFix, AmnioClear, Neox100, Neox1K, AmbioDry2, Dryflex, and Amnioexcel Products.

106. MiMedx White Paper. Qualities of MiMedx PURION Processed human amnion/chorion membrane vs amniotic allografts processed by MTF.

107. MiMedx Research Report. MMP Presence in EpiFix and AmnioFix.

108. MiMedx Research Report. MMP/TIMP Activity in EpiFix.

109. Keelan, J.A., K.W. Marvin, T.A. Sato, et al., *Cytokine abundance in placental tissues: evidence of inflammatory activation in gestational membranes with term and preterm parturition.* Am J Obstet Gynecol, 1999. 181(6): p. 1530-6.

110. Xu, P., N. Alfaidy, and J.R. Challis, *Expression of matrix metalloproteinase (MMP)-2 and MMP-9 in human placenta and fetal membranes in relation to preterm and term labor.* J Clin Endocrinol Metab, 2002. 87(3): p. 1353-61.

111. MiMedx Research Report. Presence of MHC I and MHC II in Tissue Products: Competitive Analysis.

112. MiMedx Research Report. MM-RD-00021: Impacts of Terminal Sterilization on dHACM.

113. Alberts, B., A. Johnson, J. Lewis, et al., *Fibroblasts and Their Transformations: The Connective-Tissue Cell Family, in Molecular Biology of the Cell. 4th edition.* 2002, Garland Science: New York.

114. Barker, J.N., R.S. Mitra, C.E. Griffiths, et al., *Keratinocytes as initiators of inflammation.* Lancet, 1991. 337(8735): p. 211-4.

115. Alberts, B., A. Johnson, J. Lewis, et al., *Blood Vessels and Endothelial Cells, in Molecular Biology of the Cell. 4th edition.* 2002, Garland Science: New York.

116. Prior, B.M., H.T. Yang, and R.L. Terjung, *What makes vessels grow with exercise training?* J Appl Physiol (1985), 2004. 97(3): p. 1119-28.

117. Yoo, S.Y. and S.M. Kwon, *Angiogenesis and its therapeutic opportunities.* Mediators Inflamm, 2013. 2013: p. 127170.

118. Rensen, S.S., P.A. Doevendans, and G.J. van Eys, *Regulation and characteristics of vascular smooth muscle cell phenotypic diversity.* Neth Heart J, 2007. 15(3): p. 100-8.

119. Gerthoffer, W.T., *Mechanisms of vascular smooth muscle cell migration.* Circ Res, 2007. 100(5): p. 607-21.

120. Caplan, A.I., *All MSCs are pericytes?* Cell Stem Cell, 2008. 3(3): p. 229-30.

121. Sasaki, M., R. Abe, Y. Fujita, et al., *Mesenchymal stem cells are recruited into wounded skin and contribute to wound repair by transdifferentiation into multiple skin cell type.* J Immunol, 2008. 180(4): p. 2581-7.

122. Mendez, J.J., M. Ghaedi, D. Steinbacher, et al., *Epithelial cell differentiation of human mesenchymal stromal cells in decellularized lung scaffolds.* Tissue Eng Part A, 2014. 20(11-12): p. 1735-46.

123. Schmidt-Lucke, C., F. Escher, S. Van Linthout, et al., *Cardiac migration of endogenous mesenchymal stromal cells in patients with inflammatory cardiomyopathy.* Mediators Inflamm, 2015. 2015: p. 308185.

124. Marquez-Curtis, L.A. and A. Janowska-Wieczorek, *Enhancing the migration ability of mesenchymal stromal cells by targeting the SDF-1/CXCR4 axis.* Biomed Res Int, 2013. 2013: p. 561098.

125. Farshdousti Hagh, M., M. Noruzinia, Y. Mortazavi, et al., *Different Methylation Patterns of RUNX2, OSX, DLX5 and BSP in Osteoblastic Differentiation of Mesenchymal Stem Cells.* Cell J, 2015. 17(1): p. 71-82.

126. Davey, G.C., S.B. Patil, A. O'Loughlin, et al., *Mesenchymal stem cell-based treatment for microvascular and secondary complications of diabetes mellitus.* Front Endocrinol (Lausanne), 2014. 5: p. 86.

127. Gu, W., L. Song, X.M. Li, et al., *Mesenchymal stem cells alleviate airway inflammation and emphysema in COPD through down-regulation of cyclooxygenase-2 via p38 and ERK MAPK pathways.* Sci Rep, 2015. 5: p. 8733.

128. Izadpanah, R., C. Trygg, B. Patel, et al., *Biologic properties of mesenchymal stem cells derived from bone marrow and adipose tissue.* J Cell Biochem, 2006. 99(5): p. 1285-97.

129. Zuk, P.A., M. Zhu, P. Ashjian, et al., *Human adipose tissue is a source of multipotent stem cells.* Mol Biol Cell, 2002. 13(12): p. 4279-95.

130. Dimarino, A.M., A.I. Caplan, and T.L. Bonfield, *Mesenchymal stem cells in tissue repair.* Front Immunol, 2013. 4: p. 201.

131. Gunsilius, E., G. Gastl, and A.L. Petzer, *Hematopoietic stem cells.* Biomed Pharmacother, 2001. 55(4): p. 186-94.

132. Gessner, A., K. Mohrs, and M. Mohrs, *Mast cells, basophils, and eosinophils acquire constitutive IL-4 and IL-13 transcripts during lineage differentiation that are sufficient for rapid cytokine production.* J Immunol, 2005. 174(2): p. 1063-72.

133. Aumailley, M. and B. Gayraud, *Structure and biological activity of the extracellular matrix.* J Mol Med (Berl), 1998. 76(3-4): p. 253-65.

134. Gelse, K., E. Poschl, and T. Aigner, *Collagens--structure, function, and biosynthesis.* Adv Drug Deliv Rev, 2003. 55(12): p. 1531-46.

135. Kühn, K., *The Classical Collagens: Types I, II, and III, in Structure and Function of Collagen Types*, R. Maynes and R.E. Burgeson, Editors. 1987, Academic Press, Inc.: Orlando, FL.

136. Glanville, R.W., *Type IV Collagen, in Structure and Function of Collagen Types*, R. Maynes and R.E. Burgeson, Editors. 1987, Academic Press, Inc.: Orlando, FL.

137. Amenta, P.S., S. Gay, A. Vaheri, et al., *The extracellular matrix is an integrated unit: ultrastructural localization of collagen types I, III, IV, V, VI, fibronectin, and laminin in human term placenta.* Coll Relat Res, 1986. 6(2): p. 125-52.

138. Sakai, L.Y., D.R. Keene, N.P. Morris, et al., *Type VII collagen is a major structural component of anchoring fibrils.* J Cell Biol, 1986. 103(4): p. 1577-86.

139. Shuttleworth, C.A., *Type VIII collagen.* Int J Biochem Cell Biol, 1997. 29(10): p. 1145-8.

140. van der Rest, M. and R. Mayne, *Type IX collagen proteoglycan from cartilage is covalently cross-linked to type II collagen.* J Biol Chem, 1988. 263(4): p. 1615-8.

141. Shen, G., *The role of type X collagen in facilitating and regulating endochondral ossification of articular cartilage.* Orthod Craniofac Res, 2005. 8(1): p. 11-7.

142. Eyre, D., *Collagen of articular cartilage.* Arthritis Res, 2002. 4(1): p. 30-5.

143. Nimni, M.E., *Collagen: structure, function, and metabolism in normal and fibrotic tissues.* Semin Arthritis Rheum, 1983. 13(1): p. 1-86.

144. van der Rest, M. and R. Garrone, *Collagen family of proteins.* FASEB J, 1991. 5(13): p. 2814-23.

145. Buehler, M.J., *Nature designs tough collagen: explaining the nanostructure of collagen fibrils.* Proc Natl Acad Sci U S A, 2006. 103(33): p. 12285-90.

146. James, R., G. Kesturu, G. Balian, et al., *Tendon: biology, biomechanics, repair, growth factors, and evolving treatment options.* J Hand Surg Am, 2008. 33(1): p. 102-12.

147. Martin, R.B., D.B. Burr, and N.A. Sharkey, *Mechanical Properties of Ligament and Tendon, in Skeletal Tissue Mechanics.* 1998, Springer-Verlag: New York. p. 309-46.

148. van Zuijlen, P.P., J.J. Ruurda, H.A. van Veen, et al., *Collagen morphology in human skin and scar tissue: no adaptations in response to mechanical loading at joints.* Burns, 2003. 29(5): p. 423-31.

149. McCormick, R.J., *The flexibility of the collagen compartment of muscle.* Meat Sci, 1994. 36(1-2): p. 79-91.

150. Light, N. and A.E. Champion, *Characterization of muscle epimysium, perimysium and endomysium collagens.* Biochem J, 1984. 219(3): p. 1017-26.

151. Wang, Y., T. Azais, M. Robin, et al., *The predominant role of collagen in the nucleation, growth, structure and orientation of bone apatite.* Nat Mater, 2012. 11(8): p. 724-33.

152. Broom, N.D. and C.A. Poole, *Articular cartilage collagen and proteoglycans. Their functional interdependency.* Arthritis Rheum, 1983. 26(9): p. 1111-9.

153. Liu, X., H. Wu, M. Byrne, et al., *Type III collagen is crucial for collagen I fibrillogenesis and for normal cardiovascular development.* Proc Natl Acad Sci U S A, 1997. 94(5): p. 1852-6.

154. Wenstrup, R.J., J.B. Florer, E.W. Brunskill, et al., *Type V collagen controls the initiation of collagen fibril assembly.* J Biol Chem, 2004. 279(51): p. 53331-7.

155. Mithieux, S.M. and A.S. Weiss, *Elastin.* Adv Protein Chem, 2005. 70: p. 437-61.

156. Colognato, H. and P.D. Yurchenco, *Form and function: the laminin family of heterotrimers.* Dev Dyn, 2000. 218(2): p. 213-34.

157. Potts, J.R. and I.D. Campbell, *Structure and function of fibronectin modules.* Matrix Biol, 1996. 15(5): p. 313-20; discussion 321.

158. Birkedal-Hansen, H., W.G. Moore, M.K. Bodden, et al., *Matrix metalloproteinases: a review.* Crit Rev Oral Biol Med, 1993. 4(2): p. 197-250.

159. Vu, T.H. and Z. Werb, *Matrix metalloproteinases: effectors of development and normal physiology.* Genes Dev, 2000. 14(17): p. 2123-33.

160. Kahari, V.M. and U. Saarialho-Kere, *Matrix metalloproteinases in skin.* Exp Dermatol, 1997. 6(5): p. 199-213.

161. McCawley, L.J. and L.M. Matrisian, *Matrix metalloproteinases: they're not just for matrix anymore!* Curr Opin Cell Biol, 2001. 13(5): p. 534-40.

162. Lu, C., X.Y. Li, Y. Hu, et al., *MT1-MMP controls human mesenchymal stem cell trafficking and differentiation.* Blood, 2010. 115(2): p. 221-9.

163. Kaitu'u-Lino, T.J., K. Palmer, L. Tuohey, et al., *MMP-15 is upregulated in preeclampsia, but does not cleave endoglin to produce soluble endoglin.* PLoS One, 2012. 7(6): p. e39864.

164. Visse, R. and H. Nagase, *Matrix metalloproteinases and tissue inhibitors of metalloproteinases: structure, function, and biochemistry.* Circ Res, 2003. 92(8): p. 827-39.

165. Perrimon, N. and M. Bernfield, *Cellular functions of proteoglycans--an overview.* Semin Cell Dev Biol, 2001. 12(2): p. 65-7.

166. Saksela, O., D. Moscatelli, A. Sommer, et al., *Endothelial cell-derived heparan sulfate binds basic fibroblast growth factor and protects it from proteolytic degradation.* J Cell Biol, 1988. 107(2): p. 743-51.

167. Roughley, P.J. and E.R. Lee, *Cartilage proteoglycans: structure and potential functions.* Microsc Res Tech, 1994. 28(5): p. 385-97.

168. Iozzo, R.V., *The family of the small leucine-rich proteoglycans: key regulators of matrix assembly and cellular growth.* Crit Rev Biochem Mol Biol, 1997. 32(2): p. 141-74.

169. Geng, Y., D. McQuillan, and P.J. Roughley, *SLRP interaction can protect collagen fibrils from cleavage by collagenases.* Matrix Biol, 2006. 25(8): p. 484-91.

170. Parisuthiman, D., Y. Mochida, W.R. Duarte, et al., *Biglycan modulates osteoblast differentiation and matrix mineralization.* J Bone Miner Res, 2005. 20(10): p. 1878-86.

171. Wight, T.N., *Versican: a versatile extracellular matrix proteoglycan in cell biology.* Curr Opin Cell Biol, 2002. 14(5): p. 617-23.

172. Knox, S.M. and J.M. Whitelock, *Perlecan: how does one molecule do so many things?* Cell Mol Life Sci, 2006. 63(21): p. 2435-45.

173. Farach-Carson, M.C. and D.D. Carson, *Perlecan--a multifunctional extracellular proteoglycan scaffold.* Glycobiology, 2007. 17(9): p. 897-905.

174. Friedlander, D.R., P. Milev, L. Karthikeyan, et al., *The neuronal chondroitin sulfate proteoglycan neurocan binds to the neural cell adhesion molecules Ng-CAM/L1/NILE and N-CAM, and inhibits neuronal adhesion and neurite outgrowth.* J Cell Biol, 1994. 125(3): p. 669-80.

175. Font, B., D. Eichenberger, D. Goldschmidt, et al., *Structural requirements for fibromodulin binding to collagen and the control of type I collagen fibrillogenesis--critical roles for disulphide bonding and the C-terminal region.* Eur J Biochem, 1998. 254(3): p. 580-7.

176. Roberts, A.W., *G-CSF: a key regulator of neutrophil production, but that's not all!* Growth Factors, 2005. 23(1): p. 33-41.

177. Bendall, L.J. and K.F. Bradstock, *G-CSF: From granulopoietic stimulant to bone marrow stem cell mobilizing agent.* Cytokine Growth Factor Rev, 2014. 25(4): p. 355-67.

178. Schneider, A., H.G. Kuhn, and W.R. Schabitz, *A role for G-CSF (granulocyte-colony stimulating factor) in the central nervous system.* Cell Cycle, 2005. 4(12): p. 1753-7.

179. Hamilton, J.A. and G.P. Anderson, *GM-CSF Biology.* Growth Factors, 2004. 22(4): p. 225-31.

180. Bottner, M., C. Suter-Crazzolara, A. Schober, et al., *Expression of a novel member of the TGF-beta superfamily, growth/differentiation factor-15/macrophage-inhibiting cytokine-1 (GDF-15/MIC-1) in adult rat tissues.* Cell Tissue Res, 1999. 297(1): p. 103-10.

181. Kempf, T., A. Zarbock, C. Widera, et al., *GDF-15 is an inhibitor of leukocyte integrin activation required for survival after myocardial infarction in mice.* Nat Med, 2011. 17(5): p. 581-8.

182. Kempf, T., M. Eden, J. Strelau, et al., *The transforming growth factor-beta superfamily member growth-differentiation factor-15 protects the heart from ischemia/reperfusion injury.* Circ Res, 2006. 98(3): p. 351-60.

183. Strelau, J., M. Bottner, P. Lingor, et al., *GDF-15/MIC-1 a novel member of the TGF-beta superfamily.* J Neural Transm Suppl, 2000(60): p. 273-6.

184. Schroder, K., P.J. Hertzog, T. Ravasi, et al., *Interferon-gamma: an overview of signals, mechanisms and functions.* J Leukoc Biol, 2004. 75(2): p. 163-89.

185. Dinarello, C.A., *Biology of interleukin 1.* FASEB J, 1988. 2(2): p. 108-15.

186. Dinarello, C.A., *The biological properties of interleukin-1.* Eur Cytokine Netw, 1994. 5(6): p. 517-31.

187. Wood, L.C., P.M. Elias, C. Calhoun, et al., *Barrier disruption stimulates interleukin-1 alpha expression and release from a pre-formed pool in murine epidermis.* J Invest Dermatol, 1996. 106(3): p. 397-403.

188. Arend, W.P., M. Malyak, C.J. Guthridge, et al., *Interleukin-1 receptor antagonist: role in biology.* Annu Rev Immunol, 1998. 16: p. 27-55.

189. Martinez, F.O. and S. Gordon, *The M1 and M2 paradigm of macrophage activation: time for reassessment.* F1000Prime Rep, 2014. 6: p. 13.

190. Akdis, M., S. Burgler, R. Crameri, et al., *Interleukins, from 1 to 37, and interferon-gamma: receptors, functions, and roles in diseases.* J Allergy Clin Immunol, 2011. 127(3): p. 701-21 e1-70.

191. Schindler, R., J. Mancilla, S. Endres, et al., *Correlations and interactions in the production of interleukin-6 (IL-6), IL-1, and tumor necrosis factor (TNF) in human blood mononuclear cells: IL-6 suppresses IL-1 and TNF.* Blood, 1990. 75(1): p. 40-7.

192. Steensberg, A., C.P. Fischer, C. Keller, et al., *IL-6 enhances plasma IL-1ra, IL-10, and cortisol in humans.* Am J Physiol Endocrinol Metab, 2003. 285(2): p. E433-7.

193. Moore, K.W., R. de Waal Malefyt, R.L. Coffman, et al., *Interleukin-10 and the interleukin-10 receptor.* Annu Rev Immunol, 2001. 19: p. 683-765.

194. Cooper, A.M. and S.A. Khader, *IL-12p40: an inherently agonistic cytokine.* Trends Immunol, 2007. 28(1): p. 33-8.

195. Fixe, P. and V. Praloran, *Macrophage colony-stimulating-factor (M-CSF or CSF-1) and its receptor: structure-function relationships.* Eur Cytokine Netw, 1997. 8(2): p. 125-36.

196. Saidenberg Kermanac'h, N., N. Bessis, M. Cohen-Solal, et al., *Osteoprotegerin and inflammation.* Eur Cytokine Netw, 2002. 13(2): p. 144-53.

197. Simonet, W.S., D.L. Lacey, C.R. Dunstan, et al., *Osteoprotegerin: a novel secreted protein involved in the regulation of bone density.* Cell, 1997. 89(2): p. 309-19.

198. Manzo, A., B. Vitolo, F. Humby, et al., *Mature antigen-experienced T helper cells synthesize and secrete the B cell chemoattractant CXCL13 in the inflammatory environment of the rheumatoid joint.* Arthritis Rheum, 2008. 58(11): p. 3377-87.

199. Forssmann, U., M. Uguccioni, P. Loetscher, et al., *Eotaxin-2, a novel CC chemokine that is selective for the chemokine receptor CCR3, and acts like eotaxin on human eosinophil and basophil leukocytes.* J Exp Med, 1997. 185(12): p. 2171-6.

200. Patel, V.P., B.L. Kreider, Y. Li, et al., *Molecular and functional characterization of two novel human C-C chemokines as inhibitors of two distinct classes of myeloid progenitors.* J Exp Med, 1997. 185(7): p. 1163-72.

201. Mantovani, A., A. Sica, S. Sozzani, et al., *The chemokine system in diverse forms of macrophage activation and polarization.* Trends Immunol, 2004. 25(12): p. 677-86.

202. Robertson, M.J., *Role of chemokines in the biology of natural killer cells.* J Leukoc Biol, 2002. 71(2): p. 173-83.

203. Harada, A., N. Sekido, T. Akahoshi, et al., *Essential involvement of interleukin-8 (IL-8) in acute inflammation.* J Leukoc Biol, 1994. 56(5): p. 559-64.

204. Koch, A.E., P.J. Polverini, S.L. Kunkel, et al., *Interleukin-8 as a macrophage-derived mediator of angiogenesis.* Science, 1992. 258(5089): p. 1798-801.

205. Chupp, G.L., E.A. Wright, D. Wu, et al., *Tissue and T cell distribution of precursor and mature IL-16.* J Immunol, 1998. 161(6): p. 3114-9.

206. Polito, A.J. and D. Proud, *Epithelia cells as regulators of airway inflammation.* J Allergy Clin Immunol, 1998. 102(5): p. 714-8.

207. Deshmane, S.L., S. Kremlev, S. Amini, et al., *Monocyte chemoattractant protein-1 (MCP-1): an overview.* J Interferon Cytokine Res, 2009. 29(6): p. 313-26.

208. Yadav, A., V. Saini, and S. Arora, *MCP-1: chemoattractant with a role beyond immunity: a review.* Clin Chim Acta, 2010. 411(21-22): p. 1570-9.

209. Zlotnik, A. and O. Yoshie, *Chemokines: a new classification system and their role in immunity.* Immunity, 2000. 12(2): p. 121-7.

210. Maurer, M. and E. von Stebut, *Macrophage inflammatory protein-1*. Int J Biochem Cell Biol, 2004. 36(10): p. 1882-6.

211. von Luettichau, I., P.J. Nelson, J.M. Pattison, et al., *RANTES chemokine expression in diseased and normal human tissues.* Cytokine, 1996. 8(1): p. 89-98.

212. Gao, X. and Z. Xu, *Mechanisms of action of angiogenin.* Acta Biochim Biophys Sin (Shanghai), 2008. 40(7): p. 619-24.

213. Asahara, T., D. Chen, T. Takahashi, et al., *Tie2 receptor ligands, angiopoietin-1 and angiopoietin-2, modulate VEGF-induced postnatal neovascularization.* Circ Res, 1998. 83(3): p. 233-40.

214. Maisonpierre, P.C., C. Suri, P.F. Jones, et al., *Angiopoietin-2, a natural antagonist for Tie2 that disrupts in vivo angiogenesis.* Science, 1997. 277(5322): p. 55-60.

215. Montesano, R., J.D. Vassalli, A. Baird, et al., *Basic fibroblast growth factor induces angiogenesis in vitro.* Proc Natl Acad Sci U S A, 1986. 83(19): p. 7297-301.

216. Bragdon, B., O. Moseychuk, S. Saldanha, et al., *Bone morphogenetic proteins: a critical review.* Cell Signal, 2011. 23(4): p. 609-20.

217. Binder, D.K. and H.E. Scharfman, *Brain-derived neurotrophic factor.* Growth Factors, 2004. 22(3): p. 123-31.

218. Brouillet, S., P. Hoffmann, J.J. Feige, et al., *EG-VEGF: a key endocrine factor in placental development.* Trends Endocrinol Metab, 2012. 23(10): p. 501-8.

219. Lecouter, J., R. Lin, and N. Ferrara, *EG-VEGF: a novel mediator of endocrine-specific angiogenesis, endothelial phenotype, and function.* Ann N Y Acad Sci, 2004. 1014: p. 50-7.

220. Carpenter, G. and S. Cohen, *Epidermal growth factor.* Annu Rev Biochem, 1979. 48: p. 193-216.

221. Niswander, L. and G.R. Martin, *Fgf-4 expression during gastrulation, myogenesis, limb and tooth development in the mouse.* Development, 1992. 114(3): p. 755-68.

222. Feldman, B., W. Poueymirou, V.E. Papaioannou, et al., *Requirement of FGF-4 for postimplantation mouse development.* Science, 1995. 267(5195): p. 246-9.

223. Werner, S., K.G. Peters, M.T. Longaker, et al., *Large induction of keratinocyte growth factor expression in the dermis during wound healing.* Proc Natl Acad Sci U S A, 1992. 89(15): p. 6896-900.

224. Laron, Z., *Insulin-like growth factor 1 (IGF-1): a growth hormone.* Mol Pathol, 2001. 54(5): p. 311-6.

225. Shirakata, Y., R. Kimura, D. Nanba, et al., *Heparin-binding EGF-like growth factor accelerates keratinocyte migration and skin wound healing.* J Cell Sci, 2005. 118(Pt 11): p. 2363-70.

226. Edwards, J.P., X. Zhang, and D.M. Mosser, *The expression of heparin-binding epidermal growth factor-like growth factor by regulatory macrophages.* J Immunol, 2009. 182(4): p. 1929-39.

227. Bussolino, F., M.F. Di Renzo, M. Ziche, et al., *Hepatocyte growth factor is a potent angiogenic factor which stimulates endothelial cell motility and growth.* J Cell Biol, 1992. 119(3): p. 629-41.

228. Hwa, V., Y. Oh, and R.G. Rosenfeld, *The insulin-like growth factor-binding protein (IGFBP) superfamily.* Endocr Rev, 1999. 20(6): p. 761-87.

229. Shelton, D.L. and L.F. Reichardt, *Studies on the expression of the beta nerve growth factor (NGF) gene in the central nervous system: level and regional distribution of NGF mRNA suggest that NGF functions as a trophic factor for several distinct populations of neurons.* Proc Natl Acad Sci U S A, 1986. 83(8): p. 2714-8.

230. Ziche, M., D. Maglione, D. Ribatti, et al., *Placenta growth factor-1 is chemotactic, mitogenic, and angiogenic.* Lab Invest, 1997. 76(4): p. 517-31.

231. Meyer-Ingold, W. and W. Eichner, *Platelet-derived growth factor.* Cell Biol Int, 1995. 19(5): p. 389-98.

232. Heldin, C.H. and B. Westermark, *Mechanism of action and in vivo role of platelet-derived growth factor.* Physiol Rev, 1999. 79(4): p. 1283-316.

233. Gottlieb, A.B., C.K. Chang, D.N. Posnett, et al., *Detection of transforming growth factor alpha in normal, malignant, and hyperproliferative human keratinocytes.* J Exp Med, 1988. 167(2): p. 670-5.

234. Rappolee, D.A., D. Mark, M.J. Banda, et al., *Wound macrophages express TGF-alpha and other growth factors in vivo: analysis by mRNA phenotyping.* Science, 1988. 241(4866): p. 708-12.

235. Massague, J., *The transforming growth factor-beta family.* Annu Rev Cell Biol, 1990. 6: p. 597-641.

236. Ferrara, N., H.P. Gerber, and J. LeCouter, *The biology of VEGF and its receptors.* Nat Med, 2003. 9(6): p. 669-76.

237. MiMedx Research Report. MM-RD-00022: EpiFix and AmnioFix: Total Growth Factor Content.

238. Schultz, G.S., J.M. Davidson, R.S. Kirsner, et al., *Dynamic reciprocity in the wound microenvironment.* Wound Repair Regen, 2011. 19(2): p. 134-48.

239. Gibbons, A., *Becoming human. In search of the first hominids.* Science, 2002. 295(5558): p. 1214-9.

240. Haddad, J.J., *Cytokines and related receptor-mediated signaling pathways.* Biochem Biophys Res Commun, 2002. 297(4): p. 700-13.

241. Colobran, R., R. Pujol-Borrell, M.P. Armengol, et al., *The chemokine network. I. How the genomic organization of chemokines contains clues for deciphering their functional complexity.* Clin Exp Immunol, 2007. 148(2): p. 208-17.

242. Ozaki, K. and W.J. Leonard, *Cytokine and cytokine receptor pleiotropy and redundancy.* J Biol Chem, 2002. 277(33): p. 29355-8.

243. Grant, D.S., H.K. Kleinman, I.D. Goldberg, et al., *Scatter factor induces blood vessel formation in vivo.* Proc Natl Acad Sci U S A, 1993. 90(5): p. 1937-41.

244. Kutcher, M.E. and I.M. Herman, *The pericyte: cellular regulator of microvascular blood flow.* Microvasc Res, 2009. 77(3): p. 235-46.

245. Chow, S. and J. Liu, *Design and Analysis of Clinical Trials.* Third ed. 2014: Wiley.

246. *Good Clinical Practice Guide*, in *Collaborative Institutional Training Initiative (CITI).* 2012, University of Miami.

247. *Office for Human Research Protections (OHRP).* U.S. Department of Health & Human Services; Available from: http://www.hhs.gov/ohrp/index.html.

248. *ClinicalTrials.gov.* Available from: http://www.clinicaltrials.gov.

249. *Human Subject Regulations Decision Charts.* U.S. Department of Health & Human Services: Office for Human Research Protections (OHRP); Available from: http://www.hhs.gov/ohrp/policy/checklists/decisioncharts.html

250. *Protocol Data Element Definitions.* ClinicalTrials.gov; Available from: https://prsinfo.clinicaltrials.gov/definitions.html.

251. *Informed Consent.* U.S. Department of Health & Human Services: Office for Human Research Protections (OHRP); Available from: http://www.hhs.gov/ohrp/policy/consent/index.html.

252. *§46.116 Informed Consent Checklist - Basic and Additional Elements.* U.S. Department of Health & Human Services: Office for Human Research Protections (OHRP); Available from: http://www.hhs.gov/ohrp/policy/consentckls.html.

253. *CONSORT Checklist.* CONSORT: Transparent Reporting of Trials; Available from: http://www.consort-statement.org/checklists/view/32-consort/66-title.

254. *The CONSORT Flow Diagram.* CONSORT: Transparent Reporting of Trials; Available from: http://www.consort-statement.org/consort-statement/flow-diagram.

255. Kamel, C., L. McGahan, M. Mierzwinski-Urban, et al., *Appendix 10: Levels of Evidence (EL) for Clinical Practice Guidelines, in Preoperative Skin Antiseptic Preparations and Application Techniques for Preventing Surgical Site Infections: A Systematic Review of the Clinical Evidence and Guidelines.* 2011, Canadian Agency for Drugs and Technologies in Health: Ottawa, Canada.

256. *Levels of evidence and analyzing the literature.* N.I.H. Library; Available from: http://nihlibrary.ors.nih.gov/jw/levels_of_evidence.html.

257. Aggarwal, S. and M.F. Pittenger, *Human mesenchymal stem cells modulate allogeneic immune cell responses.* Blood, 2005. 105(4): p. 1815-22.

258. Yang, L., R.M. Froio, T.E. Sciuto, et al., *ICAM-1 regulates neutrophil adhesion and transcellular migration of TNF-alpha-activated vascular endothelium under flow.* Blood, 2005. 106(2): p. 584-92.

259. Ishida, Y., T. Kondo, A. Kimura, et al., *Absence of IL-1 receptor antagonist impaired wound healing along with aberrant NF-kappaB activation and a reciprocal suppression of TGF-beta signal pathway.* J Immunol, 2006. 176(9): p. 5598-606.

260. Petersen, A.M. and B.K. Pedersen, *The role of IL-6 in mediating the anti-inflammatory effects of exercise.* J Physiol Pharmacol, 2006. 57 Suppl 10: p. 43-51.

261. Brown, G.L., L.B. Nanney, J. Griffen, et al., *Enhancement of wound healing by topical treatment with epidermal growth factor.* N Engl J Med, 1989. 321(2): p. 76-9.

262. McNiece, I.K. and R.A. Briddell, *Stem cell factor.* J Leukoc Biol, 1995. 58(1): p. 14-22.

263. Birkedal-Hansen, H., *Proteolytic remodeling of extracellular matrix.* Curr Opin Cell Biol, 1995. 7(5): p. 728-35.

264. Spravchikov, N., G. Sizyakov, M. Gartsbein, et al., *Glucose effects on skin keratinocytes: implications for diabetes skin complications.* Diabetes, 2001. 50(7): p. 1627-35.

265. Cianfarani, F., G. Toietta, G. Di Rocco, et al., *Diabetes impairs adipose tissue-derived stem cell function and efficiency in promoting wound healing.* Wound Repair Regen, 2013. 21(4): p. 545-53.

266. Marhoffer, W., M. Stein, E. Maeser, et al., *Impairment of polymorphonuclear leukocyte function and metabolic control of diabetes.* Diabetes Care, 1992. 15(2): p. 256-60.

267. Lauer, G., S. Sollberg, M. Cole, et al., *Expression and proteolysis of vascular endothelial growth factor is increased in chronic wounds.* J Invest Dermatol, 2000. 115(1): p. 12-8.

268. Jude, E.B., R. Blakytny, J. Bulmer, et al., *Transforming growth factor-beta 1, 2, 3 and receptor type I and II in diabetic foot ulcers.* Diabet Med, 2002. 19(6): p. 440-7.

269. Nie, C., D. Yang, J. Xu, et al., *Locally administered adipose-derived stem cells accelerate wound healing through differentiation and vasculogenesis.* Cell Transplant, 2011. 20(2): p. 205-16.

270. Marston, W.A., J. Hanft, P. Norwood, et al., *The efficacy and safety of Dermagraft in improving the healing of chronic diabetic foot ulcers: results of a prospective randomized trial.* Diabetes Care, 2003. 26(6): p. 1701-5.

271. Hanft, J.R. and M.S. Surprenant, *Healing of chronic foot ulcers in diabetic patients treated with a human fibroblast-derived dermis.* J Foot Ankle Surg, 2002. 41(5): p. 291-9.

272. Veves, A., V. Falanga, D.G. Armstrong, et al., *Graftskin, a human skin equivalent, is effective in the management of noninfected neuropathic diabetic foot ulcers: a prospective randomized multicenter clinical trial.* Diabetes Care, 2001. 24(2): p. 290-5.

273. Gelfand, J.M., O. Hoffstad, and D.J. Margolis, *Surrogate endpoints for the treatment of venous leg ulcers.* J Invest Dermatol, 2002. 119(6): p. 1420-5.

274. FDA. *Guidance for Industry Chronic Cutaneous Ulcer and Burn Wounds — Developing Products for Treatment.* FDA Guidance Document 2006; Available from: http://www.fda.gov/downloads/Drugs/GuidanceComplianceRegulatoryInformation/Guidances/ucm071324.pdf.

275. Kirsner, R.S., M.L. Sabolinski, N.B. Parsons, et al., *Comparative Effectiveness of a Bioengineered Living Cellular Construct vs. a Dehydrated Human Amniotic Membrane Allograft for the Treatment of Diabetic Foot Ulcers in a Real World Setting.* Wound Repair Regen, 2015.

276. Wilcox, J.R., M.J. Carter, and S. Covington, *Frequency of debridements and time to heal: a retrospective cohort study of 312 744 wounds.* JAMA Dermatol, 2013. 149(9): p. 1050-8.

277. Medicare Claims Data.

278. Smiell, J.M., T. Treadwell, H.D. Hahn, et al., *Real-world Experience With a Decellularized Dehydrated Human Amniotic Membrane Allograft.* Wounds, 2015. 27(6): p. 158-69.

279. MiMedx White Paper. EpiFix® Value Based Purchasing for Wound Care: A Cost to Closure Analysis.

INDEX OF TERMS